The
Healing
PLATFORM

by Annie Brandt

DISCLAIMER

Neither the publisher nor the author is engaged in rendering professional advice or services to the individual reader. The ideas, procedures, and suggestions contained in the book "The Healing Platform" are not intended as a substitute for the advice and/or medical call of the reader's physician, nor is it meant to discourage or dissuade the reader from the advice of his or her physician. Moreover, anyone with chronic or serious ailments should undertake any changes to his or her personal eating and lifestyle regimen under the direct supervision of his or her physician. The phrase "Build Your Own Cure" is not intended to be a claim or a promise of medical outcome. If the reader has any questions concerning the information presented in this book, or its application to his or her particular medical profile, or if the reader has unusual medical or nutritional needs or constraints that may conflict with the advice in this book, he or she should consult his or her physician. The reader should not stop prescription medications without the advice and guidance of his or her personal physician. Neither the author, editor, nor the publisher shall be liable or responsible for any loss or damage allegedly arising from any information or suggestion in this book. Neither the author, editor, nor the publisher is responsible for your specific health condition that may require medical supervision. In no event shall the publisher, editor, Annie Brandt, their heirs or assigns or associates be liable for any damages whatsoever, including special, indirect, consequential or incidental damages or damages for loss of profits, revenue, use, or data arising out of connections with this book or the use, reliance upon or performance of any material contained in or accessed from this book or the websites www.BestAnswerforCancer. org and www.IPTforcancer.com and wwwIOICP.com.

ACKNOWLEDGEMENTS

My deepest gratitude goes out to Mary Budinger, whose support, sense of humor, and stellar editing kept me positive and excited about the finish line in this project.

Many thanks also to my friends Debbie Curtis, Eleanor Harrell, Amos Ewing, and Bill Cary who keep me going day to day with their encouragement and affection. Double grats to Debbie for the patient read-through of the book and her great suggestions.

The beautiful cover art comes from Andrea Feller, who worked with us tirelessly on many renditions until we felt it was just right. Tina Shang was the author of the Chakras chart; she took my words and created a great picture.

To old friends Ann Fonfa, Bill Gleason, Jennie Gonzalez, and Rick Hill: all long-term survivors who lit the path for me to better see that there was a way forward and a possible future ahead. And to my bosom-buddy, Connie Tamez, another breast cancer patient who walked the road less traveled side-by-side with me and is another Thriver.

To new friends Ty Bollinger, Dr. Garry Gordon, Jenny Hrbacek, Doug Kaufmann, Catie Wyman Norris, and Tony O'Donnell: thank you for the blessing of your support and endorsement. And, of course, my heartfelt respect and gratitude to the many health professionals who have supported me all these years, including but not limited to: Clothilde Canale, Dr. Leigh Erin Connealy, Dr. Rick Davis, Dr. Sean Devlin, Dr. Ted Edwards, Dr. Bob Eslinger, Dr. James and Earlene

Forsythe, Dr. Michael Galitzer, Dr. Michael and Inge Gerber, Burton Goldberg, Dr. Martha Grout, Pam Hammond, Dr. Janet Hranicky, Dr. Tony Jimenez, Dr. Ben Johnson, Dr. Gus and Beverly Kotsanis, Dr. Thom Lodi, Tom Lowe, Charlie Mann, Dr. David Minkoff, Jim Poole, Seth Quinto, Dr. Kristine Reese, Suzannah Roberts, Dr. Robert Rowen, Al Sanchez, Jr., Dr. Mary Ellen Shannon, Dr. Matthew Steinberg, Dr. Jesse Stoff, Dr. Oscar Streeter, Caroline Sutherland, Dr. Julie Taguchi, Hans Truesdell, Katharine Wales, Bradford Weeks, Martie Whittekin, Dr. Juergen Winkler, Dr. Donese Worden, and Dr. John Young.

If I have forgotten to put anyone down on paper, it is the fault of my brain and not my heart. Rest assured, you are in there.

CONTENTS

FOREWORD

I have had the honor of knowing Annie Brandt for over the past decade. She has been an inspiring figure in the field of integrative oncology and patient advocacy. I became acquainted with Annie as she assumed the role of President for the Best Answer for Cancer, a non-profit organization that supported patients diagnosed with cancer and novel integrative oncology education.

When her cancer journey started in 2001, she was immediately overwhelmed and faced with the dilemma so many cancer patients encounter: what to do when your life is on the line. She was offered the traditional mastectomy, chemotherapy, and radiation. Her mind whirled as her life was upended; she could not fathom having her breasts removed and then facing the suffering she feared would come with chemotherapy and radiation therapy. She quickly rallied her resources and started exploring other options available to her.

Her research led her to information that would forever change her life. She learned of multiple modalities and lifestyle changes that could directly treat her cancer while maintaining her quality of life. One such treatment involved the use of fractionated chemotherapy with a biological response modifier, otherwise known as IPT or IPTLD, Insulin Potentiation Targeted Low Dose therapy.

Her new found approach to her cancer led to the basis of what she now calls her "Healing Platform," which consists of holistic modalities that address the "dis-eases" in her body, mind, and spirit, and topped off with targeted cancer therapies. Because of her determination to seek out a broader approach with the help of integrative oncologists, she was found to be cancer clear in a relatively short time.

By taking the road less traveled, Annie has shown us that there is another way to find healing and health when faced with such a deadly diagnosis. Her fifteen years of survival have shown us that these healing platforms can be critically effective tools for empowering and supporting cancer patients.

Before starting her cancer journey, Annie had a career in marketing, systems engineering and environmental consulting with a variety of leading edge organizations. Her curious, innovative, and entrepreneurial spirit was birthed in these early days of her professional life. Her successes in these corporate arenas motivated her to use the skills and experiences she had to build a non-profit organization that supported and brought together both physicians and patients.

Annie believed other patients should have the option of experiencing thriving *while* surviving, so she founded Best Answer for Cancer Foundation (BAFC) in 2006. BAFC is a hybrid 501(c)3 nonprofit, comprised of a physicians group, the International Organization of Integrative Cancer Physicians, and a patient-caregiver educational group.

As a national speaker, author, educator, and non-profit visionary, Annie Brandt has helped launch a paradigm shift in the approach to cancer and to how patients should interact with their own disease. It's no secret the field of oncology needs to broaden its horizons to achieve better outcomes. Her motivational leadership and persistent vigilance has led to the education of hundreds of physicians and healthcare professionals as well as thousands of patients and patient care givers. Her enlightening story is a moving one and with it comes the wisdom and counsel of a patient who has beaten the odds of stage 4 cancer and is now considered a long term survivor... I mean THRIVER!

Learn, Live, Love and Enjoy,
Sean Devlin DO, MD(H), MS
Board Member and Director of Medical Education
International Organization of Integrative Cancer Physicians
July 20, 2016

PREFACE

"What did you do to survive?" I decided to write this book after answering that question literally thousands of times. I know what it is like to get that life-threatening diagnosis, and to be staring your mortality in the face. I know that panicked feeling, that desire to know what to do RIGHT NOW! I have talked to many, many patients on the phone for hours at a time, and I have felt good about being able to help others who find themselves at this crossroads in life. But I have always felt that I was missing an opportunity to help more people. This book is a way to share my methods and tools and experience with many.

My first tip for you: consider the issue facing you a "growth opportunity." The more positive your approach and outlook, the stronger you make your immune system and the weaker you make the disease.

This book is presented to you as an interactive tool, an invitation to take part in your own healing. It is a guide you can use to build your own Healing Platform. I hope it gives you the sense of empowerment it gave me.

Will you be 100% certain of all your choices? No. But do as much research as you can and then make an informed decision. Give your choices some time to work and be observant and vigilant, but if they are not working, don't get stubborn with your opinions. Change course: be flexible and open.

The Healing Platform has literally saved my life. And it keeps life very interesting and challenging: I am always learning something new about myself, medicine, and the world around me. Because of the Healing Platform, my life is rich beyond my imagining simply because I am alive. In 2001, my imagination as far as life expectancy goes did not extend anywhere near this far!

Is the Healing Platform an easy fix? No. I do not believe there is such a thing as an easy solution to cancer and chronic disease. We are complex beings made up of many parts and shaped by many different outside influences. That is also why I do not think there will ever be *A* cure. We are all individuals, so how can one thing work for every person? I believe there are many cures available to patients today, but those cures would be combinations of things that are pertinent to that person's physiology.

I also believe that, once you are compromised by a disease, health is a constant journey. It is not a destination you arrive at and then go back to the life you previously lived. If you think about it, the life you previously lived contained all of the ingredients that brought you to the diagnosis of disease! So I don't call myself a survivor, I call myself a Thriver. When I was walking the walk of healing, I was thriving the entire time. There was no suffering or pain, or side effects from drugs or therapy. My treatments were just another doctor's appointment: no big deal. I kept thinking, "This is cancer? I thought it was supposed to be awful."

This is why I started the Best Answer for Cancer Foundation, and why I wrote this book. It is my desire that every patient of cancer and chronic disease experience "thriving while surviving" and become Thrivers themselves.

This is my gift to you and your journey.

All profits from the sale of this book will be donated to Best Answer for Cancer Foundation.

If you find a product(s) that has been vetted in this book you wish to purchase, Best Answer for Cancer and I would appreciate you taking a moment and

1. If buying directly from a person, tell them how you heard about them!

2. Or if you're purchasing through Amazon, please use AMAZON SMILE

Program for nonprofits to receive a small percentage of any/all sales using this link: www.amazon.com/ch/20-5469118. Keep us handy for all your shopping!

Amazon Smile

Shop at AmazonSmile and Amazon will make a donation to: Best Answer for Cancer Foundation

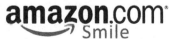

CHAPTER I

Been Here, Done This

I am alive today against all odds, according to my doctors. I am a person who has been given a potential death sentence at least four times, and I have managed and triumphed each time.

I am writing this book at the request of my family, friends, and associates so others can benefit from what I have had to learn the hard way. When you get sick, people tend to chalk that up to bad luck. But the medical community has known for a long time now that a myriad of factors often have been in play by the time the diagnosis is made: nutritional deficiencies, environmental and epigenetic stressors, emotional and psychological issues, and physical traumas. These combine to make a "stew"—a perfect storm—that breeds chronic diseases, including cancer. This book will help you identify the "stew" of ingredients in *your* own life that can lead—or has already led—to cancer and chronic disease.

Cancer doesn't start the day your doctor says, "I'm sorry, it's cancer." Cancer and other chronic illnesses merely rear their heads high enough one day so we can see them. Like the tip of the iceberg, their foundations are almost always years in the making. To understand that is to understand how to begin to take control and change your life. I call that process the *creation of a whole-being healing platform.*

By the end of this book, you will have the knowledge of how you can set up your own Healing Platform.

The whole-being Healing Platform™ is a sturdy foundation of programs, practices, products, and therapies that work together to heal the whole being. I say whole being because conventional medicine tends to see us as a disconnected bag of bones. There is one doctor for your heart, one for your lungs, one for your feet… and they all look at us from our neck down. But atop our shoulders sits the all-important key to cancer: our brain and our spiritual connection to our thoughts and feelings. Our thoughts, feelings, and interpretations of life's events are as much a part of the cancer etiology as are our genetics, our circulating tumor cells, and our white blood cell count. Our minds and our bodies *are* connected.

When conventional medicine's standard of care includes treating the whole being, I believe we will see a dramatic turnaround in cancer survival rates. Whole being treatment is especially important for later stage cancers. Until then, those of us who want to be thrivers need to create our own Healing Platform.

So let's get started!

CHAPTER II
The Cancer Personality

*C*ancer patients usually have more in common than the disease or their genetic makeup. Usually there is a set of personality traits so common to cancer patients that it is called "The Cancer Personality."

For example, a 1991 Australian study of 600 people diagnosed with colorectal cancer found they were significantly more likely to show "the elements of denial and repression of anger and of other negative emotions...the external appearance of 'nice' or 'good' person, a suppression of reactions which may offend others, and the avoidance of conflict."[1]

This concept isn't new, but is rarely discussed or related to patients. It's importance in whole-being treatment is a great starting point to understand how to start your healing journey. I began here because, when I read about the Cancer Personality and saw how closely it related to me, I knew that here was something that was fundamental to the disease. Here was something that *had* to change in order for me to stop supporting and feeding the disease. Here was something I could do myself, right away.

One of the original and most highly-regarded pioneers in the field of integrative cancer treatment, W. Douglas Brodie, M.D., of Nevada, explored the cancer personality in great depth. Although

---

1 Kune GA, Kune S et al. Personality as a risk factor in large bowel cancer: data from the Melbourne Colorectal Cancer Study. *Psychol Med.* 1991 Feb;21(1):29-41. http://www.ncbi.nlm.nih.gov/pubmed/2047503

there are more recent studies about the cancer personality, these fundamental traits were well explained by him, and they still represent a common thread in the field. Dr. Brodie said suppressed anger is the most common emotional feature of cancer patients. Here are some of his thoughts on the subject:

The Cancer Personality: Its Importance in Healing

by Dr. W. Douglas Brodie

Evidence of a relationship between cancer and personality type has existed for centuries. Going back in history to the second century AD, Galen, a Greek physician famous for his astute observations of patients and for his accurate descriptions of diseases, noted that women with breast cancer frequently had a tendency to be melancholic.

In dealing with many thousands of cancer patients over the past 28 years, it has been my observation that there are certain personality traits which are rather consistently present in the cancer-susceptible individual. These characteristics are as follows:

1. Being highly conscientious, dutiful, responsible, caring, hardworking, and usually of above average intelligence.

2. Exhibiting a strong tendency toward carrying other people's burdens and toward taking on extra obligations, often "worrying for others."

3. Having a deep-seated need to make others happy, tending to be "people pleasers." Having a great need for approval.

4. Often having a history of lack of closeness with one or both parents, sometimes, later in life, resulting in lack of closeness with spouse or others who would normally be close.

5. Harboring long-suppressed toxic emotions, such as anger, resentment and/or hostility. Typically the cancer-susceptible individual internalizes such emotions and has great difficulty expressing them.

6. Reacting adversely to stress, often becoming unable to cope adequately with such stress. Usually experiencing an especially damaging event about 2 years before the onset of detectable cancer. The patient is unable to cope with this traumatic event or series of events, which comes as a "last straw" on top of years of suppressed reactions to stress.

7. Showing an inability to resolve deep-seated emotional problems and conflicts, usually arising in childhood, often even being unaware of their presence.

Typical of the cancer-susceptible personality, as noted above, is the long-standing tendency to suppress "toxic emotions," particularly anger. Usually starting in childhood, this individual has held in his/her hostility and other unacceptable emotions. More often than not, this feature of the affected personality has its origins in feelings of rejection by one or both parents. Whether these feelings or rejection are justified or not, it is the perception of rejection that matters, and this results in a lack of closeness with the "rejecting" parent or parents, followed later in life by a similar lack of closeness with spouses and others with whom close relationships would normally develop. Those at higher risk for cancer tend to develop feelings of loneliness as a result of their having been deprived of affection and acceptance earlier in life, even if this is merely their own perception. These people have a tremendous need for approval and acceptance, developing a very high sensitivity to the needs of others while suppressing their own emotional needs.

These good folks become the "caretakers" of the world, showing great compassion and caring for others, and going out of their way to look after the needs of others. They are very reluctant to accept help from others, fearing that it may jeopardize their role as caretakers or that they might appear to have too much self-concern. Throughout their childhood they have typically been taught "not to be selfish," and they take this to heart as a major lifetime objective. All of this benevolence is highly commendable, of course, in our culture, but must be somehow modified in the case of the cancer patient. A distinction needs to be made here between the "care-giving" and the "care-taking" personality. There is nothing wrong with care-giving, of course, but the problem arises when the susceptible individual derives his/her entire worth, value and identity from his/her role as "caretaker." If this shift cannot be made, the patient is stuck in this role, and the susceptibility to cancer greatly increases.

As noted above, a consistent feature of those who are susceptible to cancer appears to be that they "suffer in silence," and bear their burdens without complaint. Burdens of their own as well as the burdens of others weigh heavily, often subconsciously as well as consciously, upon these people because they, through a lifetime of suppression, internalize their problems, cares and conflicts. The carefree extrovert, on the other hand, seems to be far less vulnerable to cancer than the caring introvert described above.

How one reacts to stress appears to be a major factor in the development of cancer. Most cancer patients have experienced a highly stressful event, usually about 2 years prior to the onset of detectable disease. This traumatic event is often beyond the patient's control, such as the loss of a loved one, loss of a business, job, home, or some other major disaster. The typical cancer victim has lost the ability to cope with these extreme events, because his/her coping mechanism lies in his/her ability to control the environment. When this control is lost, the patient has no other way to cope.

Major stress, as we have seen, causes suppression of the immune system, and does so more overwhelmingly in the cancer-susceptible individual than in others. Thus personal tragedies and excessive levels of stress appear to combine with the underlying personality described above to bring on the immune deficiency which allows cancer to thrive.

W. Douglas Brodie, M.D., (1925–2005).
© 2001 W. Douglas Brodie, MD, 601 West Moana Lane, Ste. 3, Reno, NV 89509
Reprinted with permission.

A friend of mine who overcame an autoimmune disease said that she was told early on by her colonic therapist and a nutritionist that she had to get in touch with her heart—her feelings—if she wanted to overcome her disease. Here is what she recently wrote me:

> I couldn't even comprehend what they were telling me. What did they mean by 'get out of my head?' Come on, the heart just pumps blood. It's the brain that makes thoughts and of course I am in touch with my brain. It was my brain by which I had made a successful career, not my heart. I laugh now to think back how rigid I was and how bloody hard it was to understand such a basic concept. I had absolutely no clue how to 'get out of my head.' But their advice was right on. Thanks to books like *A Course in Miracles* and learned friends, I gained many life-saving pearls of wisdom. And I came to appreciate how powerfully the mind can alter our physical properties. Unfortunately, doctors are not trained to teach this aspect of healing. It will take someone like you, Annie, to teach the patients—and the doctors—how to get beyond the needle/drug paradigm and treat the whole being.

After reading about these traits, I realized they all described me. I was astounded. How could a stranger have described me so well? But I also realized I was not alone. And I realized I could do something about this.

Developing a Cancer Personality

I was born in a small town in Wisconsin, the third of four children in a middle-class family, and spent the first 14 years of my life playing sports, camping, raising rabbits, and catching frogs and turtles.

Sounds wholesome, but our family also had a toxic secret that was really no secret at all: my mother was an alcoholic. She loved us, but I frequently felt abandoned and overlooked. I had twin sisters thirteen months older than me and the long-awaited baby brother five years behind me. My father was too busy working during the week and sobering Mom up on the weekends to give any of us much attention, but when he did it was typically to my over-achieving sisters. I always felt that I was struggling to keep up.

"More often than not, this feature of the affected person-
ality has its origins in feelings of rejection by one or both
parents."

—Brodie

I tried to get attention by being "little miss everything-is-just-fine" and "little miss fix-it." Mom knew she could always count on me to help her, or to make her feel better. I got approval from Dad for keeping Mom calm and approval from Mom for being there for her. Yet, at the same time, it seemed as if they were not there to care for me, and children want to be cared for.

"Exhibiting a strong tendency toward carrying other peo-
ple's burdens and toward taking on extra obligations, often
'worrying for others.'"

—Brodie

My mother quit drinking on my dad's promise that we would leave Wisconsin. We then moved to St. Louis, and life became a little more stable and cosmopolitan, but still fraught with emotion and uncertainty. I was constantly looking for approval and feeling that I wasn't getting it. For example, I tried out for cheerleading but did not make the squad. I came home and told my parents about it, crying, and it was as if they never heard me, never saw that I was crying. They proceeded to talk about how my sister just got an A on a test. I was always trying to shine in my parents' eyes, but was outshone by my sisters who were much more studious than I, and by my little brother who could do no wrong just because he was the baby and the only boy. No matter what I did, it seemed to me I was ignored, overlooked, or even verbally abused.

Many times I would try to help my father on the weekend around the house; he would ask for a certain tool and when I could not find it, he told me I was stupid. Or I would be given a task to do and would be criticized about my work. I found myself increasingly frustrated and angry, and I spent most of my time at home alone in my room writing in my diary in an effort to vent my emotions.

"Harboring long-suppressed toxic emotions, such as anger, resentment, and/or hostility. Typically the cancer-susceptible individual internalizes such emotions and has great difficulty expressing them."
—Brodie

It may seem as if my parents picked on me, and I may have thought so at the time. What I later learned in therapy, however, was that I probably brought much of that on myself. I projected this "everything is just fine" attitude. My parents thought they did not have to worry about sunny, calm me. The very behavior that I used to hopefully get Atta Girl pats on the back, back-fired because I remember getting very little attention and most of it negative when I did not perform. And ironically, the "everything is fine" modus operandi is also the cancer patient's personality trait.

Looking back, it seems that I spent my childhood and young adulthood trying to be noticed, to succeed, to gain approval, and failing, only to feel resentment and sorrow that I then suppressed. This pattern continued until I got sick.

"Having a deep-seated need to make others happy, tending to be 'people pleasers.' Having a great need for approval."
—Brodie

Since I got diagnosed with cancer in my left breast, I have discovered that Dr. Brodie and others have been able to statistically connect emotions and psychological aspects with different diseases. This was all news to me but it certainly made a lot of sense when I read in Louise Hay's book, *You Can Heal Your Life*, that disease of the left breast was connected with "Feeling unloved, refusal to nourish oneself. Putting everyone else first."

Your Mission

Step 1. Go back through your childhood and identify events and your reaction to those events that helped develop your cancer personality. Write them down.

_____

_____

_____

_____

_____

_____

_____

_____

_____

_____

_____

Step 2. Check the characteristics below that apply to you of Dr. Brodie's psychological profile of cancer and then think about what events, patterns, or trends in your life may fit in with the points he makes.

a. Being highly conscientious, dutiful, responsible, caring, hard-working, and usually of above average intelligence.

_____

_____

_____

_____

_____

_____

b. Exhibiting a strong tendency toward carrying other people's burdens and toward taking on extra obligations, often "worrying for others."

_____

_____

_____

_____

_____

c. Having a deep-seated need to make others happy, tending to be "people pleasers." Having a great need for approval.

_____

_____

_____

_____

_____

_____

d. Often having a history of lack of closeness with one or both parents, sometimes, later in life, resulting in lack of closeness with spouse or others who would normally be close.

_____

_____

_____

_____

_____

_____

e. Harboring long-suppressed toxic emotions, such as anger, resentment and/or hostility. Typically, the cancer-susceptible individual internalizes such emotions and has great difficulty expressing them.

_____

_____

_____

_____

_____

_____

f. Reacting adversely to stress, often becoming un-able to cope adequately with such stress. Usually experiencing an especially damaging event about 2 years before the onset of detectable cancer. The patient is unable to cope with this traumatic event or series of events, which comes as a "last straw" on top of years of suppressed reactions to stress.

_____

_____

_____

_____

_____

g. Showing an inability to resolve deep-seated emotional problems and conflicts, usually arising in childhood, often even being unaware of their presence.

_____

_____

_____

_____

_____

_____

_____

CHAPTER III

Young Life in the Fast Lane

fter college in southwestern Missouri, I ended up in a minor secretarial position with Anheuser-Busch in St. Louis. The "King of Beers" was one of corporate America's "Boys Clubs." In our whole division, there was not one woman in management. I decided it was time to break into the club. I wanted to break the glass ceiling that held most women back in the era of the late '70s, early '80s. I was going to succeed!

Within two years, my division Vice President created a job especially for me called Market Research Specialist. In this position, I got to investigate different business options for our Division, including the purchase of other companies. I researched, and was involved in the purchase of a bakery goods company in Minneapolis. I was then assigned the task of finding a computer system to automate this company. I did the research, found it, and the division management agreed with my ideas. Then I was asked to install the computer system, get it up and running, and train their personnel. It was a fun challenge, and it was great when I completed it with flying colors! Approval for my work was widespread, and I felt great.

After I completed that assignment, I got a job offer from Datapoint, the computer company I had chosen to solve the bakery goods client's needs. I accepted the Market Support Representative position. The computer industry at the time was known as a man's field. I now had several years of big-time accomplishments and approvals under my belt. My confidence was growing.

I transferred with Datapoint to the exciting city of Dallas, Texas, in 1981 as a Computer Systems Engineer in the height of the big oil boom in Texas. Two years later, my husband and I got divorced because he thought the word "fidelity" applied only to savings and loan operations. I was still dealing with the shock, betrayal, and abandonment when I got caught in a layoff as the computer industry began to downsize in 1985. Now my profession had betrayed and abandoned me. That's two emotional shocks in a matter of 2 years.

I got a new job and relocated to San Antonio, Texas, still in the computer field, this time with Digital Equipment Corporation (DEC). It was in a junior position in marketing/software support so I was back working my way up the ladder and gaining approval from the Good Ol' Boys. In the next three years, I had three promotions. By 1989, I had worked my way up to the top field software position. In 1990, I got promoted to a corporate division. In my area of expertise, there were only 12 of us, world-wide. We consulted with Fortune 100/500 companies, at the director level and above, building global information networks. I was transferred back to Dallas, bought a beautiful mini-castle of a house, drove a company car, and had a good expense account. I had "arrived!"

I also had survived my share of corporate knives in my back. Although my career was none the worse for them, my heart paid a price. Post-divorce, my new attempts at romance failed, often because the guy was unfaithful. I didn't know then what I do know, that unfaithfulness isn't about me, it's about the other person—their commitment issues, their ability to be honest with themselves and others. I tended to bury the sense of betrayal and abandonment and paint the relationships bright. After all, a successful person at work should be equally successful in love, right?

I was mostly raised with good, balanced meals—even with Mom's alcoholism. However, when I left home and went out on my own, things went downhill. I was too busy to eat right so fast food on the run was frequent. I drank alcohol and smoked cigarettes. I stayed up late. I worked very long hours because it was necessary to get ahead. I played hard to let off tension. I never worried about my health; sickness was for others. *It would not happen to me.* I was skating on the surface of life and having a great time—oblivious to the stage I had set for cancer.

I stopped smoking in 1985, but my health seemed to get worse. In 1986, when I got my first promotion in DEC, I also got allergies. I know now that allergies are a symptom that the immune system has been compromised, but I didn't know it then. I tried shots, but I was allergic to everything that grew, so the shots would make my whole arm or leg swell up. I ended up on heavy doses of oral medicines.

In 1987, I was diagnosed with an intestinal allergy to beef. The following year, I got gastritis, an inflammation of the intestinal tract. In 1989, I made the really intelligent decision that I needed breast implants and some dental work. So I introduced two hefty toxins into my already weakened body: silicone and heavy metals in the dental work. In 1990, when moved to Dallas, my busy lifestyle picked up even more. I was living the good life: lots of travel, nice restaurants, rich food, and late nights. I was working 60-80 hours/week, and still playing hard.

Your Mission

Think about the occurrences, places, and people that reinforced the dis-ease in your life. Try not to cover it up emotionally, to 'make it come out right.' This is a form of self-abuse, because deep inside, we KNOW it was not all right. It is important in this process that we expose all of the wounds so that we can set about healing them.

_____

_____

_____

_____

_____

_____

_____

_____

_____

_____

_____

_____

_____

_____

_____

_____

_____

_____

_____

_____

_____

_____

_____

CHAPTER IV

Falling into the Abyss

Chronic Fatigue Immune Dysfunction Syndrome (Myalgic Encephalomyelitis)

By 1992, I had a serious relationship with a man I loved and admired, and we had talked of marriage. I had many friends, great pets, and the relationship with my parents was loving and approving.

All was right with my world. Then in an instant, it came crashing down.

I was in Boston at a World Conference for DEC talking to a Vice President of Kodak about an international network solution for his company. I paused to take a breath in the middle of a sentence and then couldn't remember the rest of my thought. Worse than that, I looked at this man I had just spent the majority of the morning with and I could not remember his name or his company! I felt a sharp stab of panic and fear. I also felt very strange physically: feverish, achy, dizzy, and nauseous. My account manager knew something was wrong. He covered for me, and we got through the awkward moment. Afterwards, he suggested that I might have the flu, so I went back to the hotel to bed and flew home the next day.

I stayed home for a few days until I felt better and then tried to go back to work. I fell asleep on my desk 45 minutes after I walked in!

I went home again for a few days. This pattern kept up for weeks. It felt like a very bad case of flu: headache, body aches, nausea, extreme fatigue, chills, fever, and mind-fog. I was so weak that some days I had to crawl to the bathroom. Several doctors and a few months later, I was finally diagnosed with Chronic Fatigue Immune Dysfunction Syndrome (CFIDS), also known as Myalgic Encephalomyelitis (ME).

Chronic Fatigue is such a misnomer to those of us that have experienced it, because it is so much more complex than that. Therefore, in this book, I will be calling it by its more acceptable name: Myalgic Encephalomyelitis (ME).

I was relieved to finally have a diagnosis. Now, I thought, I could simply take a pill and get well. So I asked the diagnosing physician what I needed. He calmly looked back at me and said, *"Well, there is nothing that we know of that will address this disease. You just have to ride it out. It may last only 6 weeks. If it lasts longer than that, it could last forever. The only things we can give you are drugs to treat the symptoms."*

I was shocked. I had been raised to believe that when you got sick, you went to the doctor, and he made you well again. Doctors were like God; they had the power of life and death, and they could "fix" you. So I took the pills for my symptoms. They not only didn't "fix" me, I actually got sicker. Each medicine came with its own set of side effects, for which I then had to get a new medicine. My monthly co-pay for this drug cocktail was $600. It had never occurred to me before that if I got sick, that doctors and the medical system might be fallible.

ME is a horrible disease. Think of how you feel during a severe case of the flu and then imagine having that flu 24/7, for years. That is ME. It can be totally incapacitating, and it was for me. I slid from the top rungs of the ladder to the basement. I was literally bedridden for 22 hours per day at first. I only had short-term disability with the company; the day my short-term disability ended was the day I got laid off—chalk that up to a third emotional trauma around the growing pile of betrayal and abandonment.

I physically still could not work, so I watched my savings disappear while I tried to get well enough to deal with the issues of selling the house, finding a new place, and moving. My boyfriend decided that he could not deal with a sick person either, which was a common reaction toward me in those days. When he met me, he fell in love with a vibrant, successful, professional woman. The abrupt change to a bedridden, chronically ill person must have been a huge shock to him. How could he reconcile a future with a sick person? Our picture of the future was what we could do together as two healthy, vibrant people, not what he could do while supporting a person physically, monetarily, and emotionally. He told me he didn't think it was going to work out anymore, and I let him go.

I did not blame him. I did not want to be with me, either. Looking at my "worth" at this point, there was not much to see. If where you lived, what you drove, and what you did for a living determined your worth, I was indeed worthless. "What do you do?" was the standard first question in a social situation. In a professional situation, your title determined the pecking order in a group and the level of respect you got.

I had always known, of course, that our society attached worth to consumer goods. I had been very good "keeping up with the Joneses." It was a rude awakening to find out that if you weren't able to obtain and possess all these things, you were essentially considered worthless and beneath notice. Sick people are pushed off the career ladder, pushed away by friends and significant others, and generally made to feel like losers. This sense of worthlessness and disapproval added another dollop of psychological trauma to my "stew."

When the unemployment ran out, I applied for Social Security Disability (SSD). Just filling out the stack of paperwork was exhausting, and emotionally and psychologically debilitating. Was I really filling out paperwork to live off the government and be declared *disabled*? Really? But I did it and sent it in. Six weeks later, I received a reply that SSD didn't consider that I was sick enough. I was in bed 20-22 hours per day. I appealed, to no avail. I applied to Supplemental Security Income (SSI) so that I could get food stamps so that I could eat. But I could not get SSI because I owned a house and a car. The government safety net wasn't designed for people like me.

There was also a great deal of skepticism from others towards my situation. ME was a very little-known disease. I got a lot of feedback that perhaps it was all in my mind, or maybe I just felt I needed a little break from working, or that if I just got out there and worked I would feel better. One doctor even told me that he thought it was female hysteria. Most of my "friends" disappeared, which added more dollops of resentment to my stew.

I started finding out anything I could about ME, which was not much in 1992. Late that year, Drs. Michael Rosenbaum and Murray Susser would publish *Solving the Puzzle of Chronic Fatigue Syndrome*. But remember there was no Google in 1992, and not that much internet for public use. For me to have found that one book would have been like finding a needle in a haystack. Even today, most of the mainstream medical community is still unfamiliar with the book's concept that ME is a disorder of the immune system involving possibly many infections.

What I did turn up was horrible: the majority of people with ME did not get over it and ended up with other auto-immune diseases such as multiple sclerosis, lupus, diabetes, and cancer. Many people did not survive. What in the world had I done wrong? Why me?

That was when I realized that conventional care was not going to fix this disease, and nobody was going to help me; I needed to figure things out for myself. I needed to heal myself.

Think about your health before you manifested the first signs of cancer. Find the signs and check below:

- ☐ allergies,
- ☐ stomach problems,
- ☐ chemical sensitivities,
- ☐ chronic bronchitis,
- ☐ high blood pressure,
- ☐ other _____

The boxes you checked was what your body was using to tell you it was having a harder and harder time maintaining balance.

Write down each of those signs separately, because next we are going to start defining the components of the platform. For each sign, write down the supplements, therapies, exercise, etc., that you did to get that symptom under control. If you used prescription medications, write those down but also note the side-effects and what you did to alleviate them.

_____

_____

_____

_____

CHAPTER V

Discovering My Healing Platform

Nutrition: My First Healing Platform Key

*A*true friend, Carol Ann, gave me a book called *The Yeast Syndrome* by William Crook, M.D. Many of the symptoms were similar to mine, and Crook speculated there might be a connection to ME, so I decided to try the yeast-free diet.

It is basically a diet of fresh foods with no sugar or yeast. No processed foods. No fast food. No shortcuts. I had to spend time and effort on my food. I had to re-nourish a depleted body. It sounds simple, but it's incredibly difficult when you are basically bed-bound with little energy. I was determined I was going to try something to help myself that made sense, something that might help repair my body. It was very difficult, physically, to manage a complicated diet, but I was determined. It meant mostly fresh meats and vegetables. And I felt a little better. It was a new idea to me that diet—what you put in your mouth—could make a difference in your body.

I now know that "you are what you eat" to a very large extent. Garbage in, garbage out (GIGO) is another way to look at it. It is essential to understand that if you take toxic foods into your body, your body will eventually become toxic. Medical schools don't teach this to doctors. TV commercials don't teach it to our kids. Yet food is fuel for the body and we need to put in the very best fuel we can.

This premise is one of the foundation stones of The Healing Platform.

Power of the Mind Over the Body:
My Second Healing Platform Key

About this time, I was able to try watching TV again. Remember, ME is like a bad flu; you cannot concentrate or make sense of things for very long, nor do you want to. So TV was out for about the first year and a half. I was in bed feeling too sick to get out from under a warm blanket that made no demands of me. When I started working with the yeast-free diet, I started feeling slightly better and that was encouraging. I made myself eat my meals out of bed, but I allowed myself to lounge on the couch. Well, there was the TV right in front of me that I hadn't been able to watch for so long.

I decided I would challenge my mind with shows, like Wheel of Fortune, Jeopardy, and PBS documentaries—television shows where the mind is forced to work. A really strange thing happened. Jeopardy did not work for me at all. I was busy trying to make sense of the answer when they would flash the next answer up. That shouldn't be happening because I was a big trivia buff. However, Wheel of Fortune, a show I did not think I would like at all because I was terrible at Scrabble, was a snap. Sometimes just one or two letters would be up on the board and I would know the answer. It appeared that the cognitive dysfunction part of ME may have rewired my brain. But clearly, I had made some progress with the brain fog and I was able to actually think and make sense of something.

Then I watched a PBS program entitled, "Bill Moyers: Healing and the Mind." This series was all about the power of the mind over the body. Moyers gave example after example of people who had overcome things or changed their lives, simply through their thoughts. As he discussed how the mind could alter what went on in the body, the light bulb went off in my head. Up until this point, I had looked at my situation from the victim point-of-view. I was so convinced I was a victim of my body and my health, and I wasn't sure if anything could help me.

Thank you Bill Moyers for my epiphany. I revisited my "little-train-that-could" attitude that I had employed most of my adult life—"I think I can, I think I can." I decided to do what I could to take control of my body through my attitude and my beliefs. I started telling myself every day that I was feeling better, that I was getting better, that I didn't ache, and that I wasn't exhausted. I was actually able to add another out-of-bed hour to my day.

Now I could spend some energy (that extra hour) trying to sell the house. I had to figure out where I could go with no money coming in and no foreseeable possibility of working. My parents came to my rescue, offering to take me to their home in Wilmington, North Carolina. They had a beach condo available where I could live for free; the only problem was that it was four stories up—no elevator. Since I no longer had a back yard, I would have to walk my dog every day, which meant going down and up daily for her and for my food.

I was really excited about living on the beach. They didn't have to twist my arm too hard. So in 1993, my parents came and moved me to North Carolina. How did I get up and down those stairs? In the beginning, on my butt using my hands and knees for leverage, stopping to rest numerous times.

I stayed with the yeast diet. Eventually, I got off all my medications and gradually got to where I could make it up and down the stairs twice a day to walk the dog.

Detox: My Third Healing Platform Key

The ocean was very healing. I think instinctively we know that the clean air and the movement of the waves are good for us. I later learned about the ozone and ionization created by the sun, the wind, and the waves (thunderstorms create the same ozone and ionization, by the way), but at the beginning I just appreciated that the air in my apartment was fresh and clean and the beauty of the beach scenery lifted my spirits. Later I discovered the ozone was neutralizing the volatile organic compounds (VOCs) in my apartment. The negative ions were removing the particulates from the air. I dropped down from 20 hours of sleep each day to 18—a huge drop for me.

Shortly after I moved to the beach, a friend of mine told me about ESSIAC® tea. ESSIAC tea came from a nurse in Canada named Rene Caisse (ESSIAC is her name spelled backwards), who got the formula from the Indians. ESSIAC tea contains four herbs, three of which are blood purifiers and one that is an anti-cancer herb. I thought I would try the tea to purify and detoxify my blood.

The ESSIAC tea actually caused a physical detoxification of sorts. And I felt a little better. I needed one less hour of sleep now, just 17 hours per day.

At first, I bought pre-mixed organic herbs from an herbalist and then brewed/steeped my own ESSIAC tea. Later on, I mixed my own organic herbs and brewed my own tea. And most recently, I learned that it takes the *roots* as well as the herbs.

The same friend who told me about ESSIAC told me about wild blue green algae, a supplemental "food" that digests at the cellular level and therefore detoxifies at the cellular level. My friend bought me a supply of the product and I tried it. Wow, what a huge difference it made, and very quickly! I dropped down to 16 hours of sleep per day. The algae I bought came from Klamath Lake, and it was sold by Cell Tech.

I was still weak and tired easily. I had to rest after any physical exertion for long periods of time, sometimes for hour, sometimes for days.

I have spent this much time writing about the ME because I believe that it is the basis upon which all my other diseases and conditions are based. To this day, it is the bane of my existence. The Chronic Fatigue part of the name is really an injustice. Yes, the fatigue is bad. However, the Immune Dysfunction Syndrome is much worse. You know that old phrase: "If Mama ain't happy, ain't nobody happy"? Well, *if the immune system ain't healthy, ain't nothin' healthy*. In some of my readings on ME, I had read that it was such a serious disease that some people could die from it. Others could get cancer or other auto-immune diseases. Well, I thought, maybe that is true for other people, but not surely not for me.

Multiple Sclerosis

A year after I had been at the beach, my doctor at the time decided he should do an MRI of the brain to help my Disability Appeal (yes, I was still trying). Evidently, ME has also shown brain lesions as one of the physical symptoms. The MRI technician gave me some contrast, did the MRI, and I went home. I did not feel well, but I thought that it was just a bad ME day. The next morning, when I got out of bed, I fell down. I had no equilibrium at all. I also got sick to my stomach. My first thought was that it was a very bad flu or a severe ME episode, so I went back to bed, assuming it would get better. However, every time I rolled over or tried to get up, I vomited. I still had no equilibrium, and after three days I also had double-vision and numbness. After nine days of vomiting, I was admitted to the hospital. It took them another four days to stop the vomiting and re-hydrate me. When they looked at my MRI, their initial suspicion was Multiple Sclerosis (MS). Testing confirmed it. But the dye they used caused me to spiral downward.

When I was released from the hospital, my parents took me into their house instead of to the apartment. I could barely walk, and needed a cane. I was wearing an eye patch, because I still could only see double. And I still had little use of one arm and one leg. I had reached a new low, and I was in despair. I vowed to myself that I would not end up in a wheelchair. I thought if that kind of downhill slide was where this was all headed, that I would walk into the garage, turn on the car, and end my life.

My doctor suggested that perhaps I had had MS the whole time and not ME. So my parents took me up to Duke University for a second opinion from one of the most recognized neurological physicians in the U.S. He confirmed that I had both. I remember thinking *"Well, you never do things by halves, do you Ann?"*

Some good did result from this diagnosis. Social Security decided that I was now sick enough to receive disability.

When I spoke to the neurologist about what came next in the treatment of the MS, he said basically the same thing the ME diagnosing physician had said. There was no cure, per se, but there were drugs to handle the symptoms and slow the progression of the disease. I quickly determined that I could not afford the drugs. He cautioned me that I had the progressive/aggressive MS and that I would probably be in a wheelchair very quickly (within six months to one year) and that it would most likely be fatal. I was only 39.

Spirituality: My Fourth Healing Platform Key

I worked hard to make my parents believe that I was well enough to be left alone in the house. When they finally decided to take an outing, I had my suicide letter ready. I headed out to the separate garage. I had to pause to rest on the window seat near the front door, and there I broke down crying, feeling sorry for myself and saying goodbye to my dog.

This was when I heard God speak to me for the first time. A voice said, "Do not worry." My first thought was that someone had broken into the house. Then I realized that, even though it was a voice, as clear as if spoken by someone sitting next to me, it was a voice inside me. It filled the room, but it was resonating inside me. I could not tell you if it was a male or female voice, but it was a voice and I knew it was God. "I love you and will not let anything bad happen to you; you must have faith in Me." Immediately, an incredible peace and confidence came over me. However, I was so non-spiritual at the time, so naive, that I said aloud, "Okay, I'll give you six months to prove it!" I am sure God smiled at me.

I was so amazed at the experience that I decided to give in to my parents' wishes and go to their church. It was an amazing place, St. John's Episcopal in Wilmington, North Carolina. At St. John's, I found a huge, loving, happy, joyous family ready to embrace me. They encouraged me to come to The Healing Service, where they practiced Laying on of Hands to call down healing to the sufferer, whether it is physical, mental, emotional, spiritual. When I opened myself up to this practice, I actually felt warmth and movement inside me physically and spiritually. I now believe that Reiki uses the same energy source as the Laying on of Hands—the Higher Power of all of us, or God.

I did not turn anything over to God at this point, because I still did not trust Him enough to give up all control. But I was learning how to walk with Him and talk with Him.

Tweaking the Nutrition Component to Include the MS

Now I felt strengthened, supported, and comforted. But I still had to do something to fix the MS. The first thing I did was to decide that I was going to use the power of my mind and tell my body that I did not have MS, and that I was never going to have another "episode." I made that thought my Truth.

However, I still had physical weakness/imbalance, and blurred vision. Then a dear friend of my mother's (and now mine), Susan Butler, gifted me with a small soft-cover booklet called *New Hope Real Help for those who have Multiple Sclerosis,* which talked about Dr. Roy L. Swank's MS diet and offered supplements to add to the diet. The book's author, John Pageler, talked about how he used this program to take himself from being wheelchair-bound to playing tennis again. It is now hard to find this book, but I did locate it on Amazon recently.

I immediately got Dr. Swank's book and got on the diet. It was not much different than the yeast-free diet, but there were some changes that I made. I always have to balance new ideas with what I know works for the ME. I bought all the supplements that John Pageler recommended. There were many supplements to repair the myelin sheath of the brain, to strengthen all the neurotransmitters and neurological pathways, to strengthen and boost the immune system. I started taking about 30-60 pills each day and I noticed a quick response from all of these. The double and blurred vision went away; the numbness, lack of balance and dizziness started abating. Within six months, instead of being in a wheelchair as the doctor had predicted, I was functioning fairly normally.

Exercise: My Fifth Healing Platform Key

The neurologist told me that exercise would be helpful to MS, and helpful with the lack of balance and dizziness. Unfortunately, this is where I ran into a big dilemma: because of the ME, I had no energy reserves. A normal person can rest and recharge these reserves; a person with ME, if they run the reserves down, has to rest for days at the very least to build up their strength again. If a person with ME stands on their feet for too long, their blood pressure drops. However, I was determined. So, I took my little dog, Tina Turner (all black and great legs ☺), for gentle walks around the neighborhood with my mom. I always stopped at the first sign of fatigue; I never taxed myself. In this way, I gradually got rid of the numbness and dizziness.

Thanks to these changes and additions, within six months of my ultimatum to God, I was symptom-free, as long as I stayed stress-free. I was able to move back to my beach apartment and was able to go up and down the four flights of stairs with periodic rests. I have never had another big episode, just occasionally small episodes and minor symptoms when the stress levels get too high or when I exert myself too much physically.

I had no idea what still lay ahead of me.

Mitral Valve Prolapse

In 1995, I had no sooner gotten the MS under control when I was diagnosed with a heart condition in which the valve that separates the upper and lower chambers of the left side of the heart does not close properly. They call this Mitral Valve Prolapse. Luckily, the doctor said we could hold off on any medication. There was nothing I could do for this one except to use my mind to "tell" my heart that it was okay and then work to stay healthy.

Multiple Chemical Sensitivity (MCS)

My beach condo was destroyed in 1996 after hits from Hurricanes Bertha and Fran. I stayed with my parents until they bought a new investment condo property, and they helped me move in. It was a brand new property. I did not realize what I was walking into: a highly toxic mix of Volatile Organic Compounds (VOCs).

According to the EPA[2]:

Volatile organic compounds (VOCs) are emitted as gases from certain solids or liquids. VOCs include a variety of chemicals, some of which may have short- and long-term adverse health effects. Concentrations of many VOCs are consistently higher indoors (up to ten times higher) than outdoors. VOCs are emitted by a wide array of products numbering in the thousands.

Organic chemicals are widely used as ingredients in household products. Paints, varnishes and wax all contain organic solvents, as do many cleaning, disinfecting, cosmetic, degreasing and hobby products. Fuels are made up of organic chemicals. All of these products can release organic compounds while you are using them, and, to some degree, when they are stored.

EPA's Office of Research and Development's "Total Exposure Assessment Methodology (TEAM) Study" (Volumes I through IV, completed in 1985) found levels of about a dozen common organic pollutants to be 2 to 5 times higher inside homes than outside, regardless of whether the homes were located in rural or highly industrial areas.

The day I moved my furniture in, I got a blinding headache. I felt dizzy and my head felt like it was full of wool. My eyes started watering, and my vision got blurry. Worst of all, I could feel my throat closing up. I started having difficulty breathing. Before an hour had passed, I had to leave.

I was diagnosed with Multiple Chemical Sensitivity (MCS). Clinical ecologists generally define MCS as an adverse reaction to potentially

---

2 https://www.epa.gov/indoor-air-quality-iaq/volatile-organic-compounds-impact-indoor-air-quality

toxic chemicals in air, food, or water, at concentrations generally accepted as harmless to the bulk of the population.[3]

I could not go into any environments that had chemicals in them. This meant department stores, hardware stores, new houses, the detergent isle of the grocery store, and places where people used perfumes and colognes. In other words, it meant I could not go anywhere; even my home was toxic.

MCS led me to explore "detoxifying" not only my body but also my environment in the house and everywhere else I went.

I removed all cleaning materials, candles, perfumes, aerosols, etc., wanting to eliminate as many of the VOCs as possible. I stopped using scented cleansers and detergents, reverting to vinegar and other less toxic cleaners. Also I learned that the paints, carpets, furniture, etc. in most homes will off-gas for up to 12 years. About the time it stops releasing chemicals, people figure it is time to "refresh" their paint, carpet, and furniture, and thus the toxic cycle starts over again.

Below is a chart on the everyday harmful chemicals in our air and their effects on us and those around us.

So if you are wondering what symptoms you might have from using a typical VOC paint, go to the Paints line under SOURCES. The yellow arrows in the chart point down to benzene, trichloroethylene, and carbon tetrachloride.

If you are wondering what chemicals in your environment might be causing headaches, go to Headaches in the SYMPTOMS section and follow the green arrows up. The green arrows point to seven of the common gasses on the list.

What do the red dotted lines and arrows mean? Asthma and allergies are usually the first things that show up when the immune system is compromised. On the chart, follow the red dotted line over to the first green arrow to chloroform and then look above and you see that chloroform is found in carpeting, drapes, and upholstery.

3 Dr. William J Rea, et all; Confirmation of chemical sensitivity by means of double-blind inhalant challenge of toxic volatile chemicals, *Clinical Ecology*, Volume VI, number 3.

SOURCES AND SYMPTOMS
OF
COMMON *GASeous* INDOOR AIR POLLUTANTS
This Chart Compliments of: Healthy Spaces, LLC (512-342-8181)

SOURCES

- Paints
- Carpets-Drapes
- Upholstery
- Tobacco Smoke
- Cleaning Supplies
- Plywood-Particle Board-Cabinets-Paneling
- Furniture
- Office Dividers
- Wall Paper
- Gas Burners-Furnaces
- Glues

COMMON GASES → Benzene | Ammonia | Chloroform | Formaldehyde | Benzopyrene | Hydrocarbons | Trichloroethylene | Carbon Tetrachl

SYMPTOMS

- Headaches
- Breathing Distress
- Respiratory Problems
- Eye Irritation
- Skin Irritation
- Fatigue
- Cancer
- Nose Bleeds
- Sinus Problems
- Asthma
- Dizziness
- Drowsiness
- Respiration Irritation
- Memory Loss
- Depression
- Gynecological Prob.
- Lung Cancer

(Gases from individual products vary somewhat from manufacturer to manufacturer)

NOTE: Just recently, I checked back with my sources and the chemicals benzopyrene, hydrocarbons, and trichloroethylene have all been labeled as "probable" in the carcinogen category. The two "probable" carcinogens labeled in the table above—chloroform and carbon tetrachloride—are now categorized as carcinogens.

I had help in learning about the toxicity that is part of our modern lifestyle. A girlfriend introduced me to a very good looking fellow who was way ahead of me when it came to "going green." He was a type 1 diabetic, yet he was on very little medication. He was a green designer/builder. We hit it off famously from the start and he became my boyfriend, and eventually my husband.

Additions to my Detox Key

Together, he and I bought a HEPA filter to take care of particulates, and we outfitted the new apartment with some plants that were known to filter VOCs, including ivy, mother-in-law's tongue, dieffenbachia, and rubber plants. The air in the apartment killed three sets of plants (Lowe's kept replacing them for free) before I could stay in the apartment for a whole day. It took several weeks of filtering before I was able to move in. Even then, I had to keep the windows open so that fresh air could come in. Ozone is found in fresh air, and ozone is known to convert VOCs to harmless combinations of carbon dioxide and water, substances that are useful to us.

I then bought an ionizer to put negative ions in my home (similar to the natural effect of being at the ocean), because I had learned about the way that negative ions would cause particulates to fall out of the air. This is also why the air smells so fresh after a thunderstorm; the action of the wind and the lightning create negative ions and ozone, which clean the particulate and bacteria out of the air. All together, they did a good job. However, I found out I could only treat one room at a time with the filter; it also used a lot of electricity and needed frequent filter changes. In addition, there was no control over how many negative ions were put into the air. It is a scientific fact that the negative ions will stick on to something: with my home, they stuck on the walls and surfaces. It looked like a grainy black dust, but you could not get it off. I had to paint over it to cover it.

In 1997, my boyfriend and I had been together for over a year, and I noticed that he was having problems gaining traction as a green builder in the Carolinas. People in that part of the country were not that environmentally aware yet. I saw people throw bags of trash out the windows of their vehicles; you would come across full baby diapers on the pristine-white sand beaches. I suggested that he consider moving his company to a more environmentally-friendly location such as Seattle, Portland, Santa Fe, or Austin. After we attended a friend's wedding in Texas and he had time to look around, he made his decision to relocate to Austin, Texas.

I was thrilled to be back in Texas. The only problem was that we rented a north-facing apartment in the middle of a cedar grove. Not only was I surrounded by trees to which I was allergic, there was toxic mold throughout the apartment. The situation overwhelmed the plants and the filter.

Shortly after moving in, I heard about a unit by a company called Alpine that *infiltrated* the air instead of filtering it. This unit would allow me to treat the whole house—up to 3,000 sq. ft. It used very little electricity, and had no filters to replace. It also eliminated toxic chemicals as well as particulates. Unlike an ionizer or an ozonator, it did not just pump out negative ions or ozone. Rather, the ions were passive and were created by radio waves, and the ozone was controlled by a computer chip to put out just .04 parts per million of ozone, the amount the EPA said was safe in indoor environments.

I found a representative in Dallas who could lend me a unit to try for a few days. The difference was amazing. The mold quickly died, the pollens did not bother me, and the unit took care of the out-gassing from the new coat of paint and new carpeting the management had installed in the apartment.

Because I found this product miraculous, and because I felt that it could help so many people, I bought a distributorship and have shared this product with many people over the last 19 years. The company has changed hands a few times and is now called Vollara. The product remains just as powerful in controlling and eliminating particulate and VOCs. It provides quality indoor air, which is essential for allowing the immune system to rest and, therefore, get stronger.

My learning curve eventually got me to the toxins found in water. It is truly scary what chemicals and chlorine by-products are in our water supply, our pools, and our lakes, rivers, and oceans. Municipal water systems, for example, do not filter out drugs so we are drinking someone else's birth control pills, or statins, or antidepressants. I learned that our skin is the largest organ of our bodies, and it is very absorbent. When we shower, we can take in more chlorine than drinking eight glasses of tap water. After discovering the dangers in water, I did more research and found a water purifier that I liked by the same company from which I got the air purifier.

I still have this company's air and water products, as well as water ionizers/alkalizers from two other companies called IonWays and LIFE Ionizers. To this day, I give credit to these products for keeping me as stable as possible.

Go back to the first time you had an illness that you had to participate in: one that the doctors could not fix with medications or medical intervention alone. Examine what you did to get well. Into which of these aspects did your participation fall? List what you tried as well as what worked—remember that what you tried and what worked can be different things.

1. Spirituality?

_____

_____

_____

_____

_____

_____

_____

_____

2. Exercise?

_____

_____

_____

_____

_____

_____

3. Detox?

_____

_____

_____

_____

_____

_____

4. Nutrition?

_____

_____

_____

_____

_____

_____

_____

5. Mind/Body?

_____

_____

_____

_____

_____

_____

_____

What else have you found?

_____

_____

_____

_____

_____

_____

_____

_____

_____

_____

_____

_____

_____

_____

_____

_____

_____

_____

_____

_____

_____

_____

_____

_____

_____

_____

_____

_____

CHAPTER VI
The Cancer Dance

I felt I was back in the real world at this point. I was in love, I was back in Texas, and my health was somewhat stable. I was still what doctors call "calendar unreliable," meaning I cannot keep to schedules very well or put forth consistent, contiguous effort. I still had episodes of ME and minor flashes of MS, and I only had about four to six hours of non-contiguous energy available to me each day. But hope springs eternal, as the saying goes. My boyfriend and I joined forces—his "green" expertise combined with my good credit and healthy financial standing. The business showcased his talents in the environmental and architectural design space. Our company was a green design/build company, and Austin was the perfect place for that, we thought.

Unfortunately, my boyfriend, while ahead of his time when it came to green design and building, wasn't savvy about the business details or customer satisfaction. We faced our first legal action within six months of moving to Austin.

We got married in 1999, and one week after the wedding got a call from the IRS. I learned my husband owed $165,000 in back taxes from before I even knew him, and now I was equally responsible for his debt. We went through a lengthy and painful "Offer in Compromise," and I ended up paying the resulting settlement to the IRS. Also shortly after the wedding, we got served with three lawsuits, one of them from our neighbor.

It was during this time that I realized my husband was abusive psychologically and emotionally.

The lawsuits continued, the work continued, the money continued to come in and go out—mostly out. Life was very stressful financially, professionally, and emotionally. It took a physical toll on my fragile health. Like most abused people, I never knew when the other shoe would drop.

Hope arrived in the form of a man who wanted to go into business with us on a work-live project in downtown Austin. Our new company, with our new partner in place, bought a full city block on the side of town that was considered the "wrong side" even though it was a mere couple of blocks from the vibrant city center. Our plan was to do a green work/live development, all condos and offices having city views. My husband was a visionary, but he was more "bleeding edge" than "leading edge." We had investors in place, and things looked exciting and wonderful, and then 9/11 happened. The investors disappeared. We held on to the property for another two and a half years before losing it completely.

I came to learn an awkward truth: my husband had married me with an eye on my money. I had a small stock portfolio and I was part of a class action lawsuit regarding silicone breast implants (which I had removed after the cancer diagnosis). My husband saw a financial future in me.

These were emotional stresses and toxins that I believe set the stage for cancer.

There is some evidence that cancer shows up two years after a traumatic event. I was diagnosed in 2001, and in 1999, we dealt with the IRS, multiple lawsuits, and I had discovered I married an abusive person. However, I think it is too simple to say that the cancer was a result of the stresses of those two years. I think that the last two years were just the icing on the cake of what had come before and the cake itself was a strong foundation of "dis-ease."

Go back two to ten years prior to your cancer diagnosis and make note of all the toxic events and people.

_____

_____

_____

_____

_____

_____

_____

Look especially close for traumatic events.

_____

_____

_____

_____

_____

Write down how you felt at the time. Did it reinforce the traits in your cancer personality? If so, which one(s)?

_____

_____

_____

_____

_____

_____

_____

_____

_____

_____

_____

_____

_____

How do you feel about it now? Have you dealt with the emotions or are they like a bruise that it still hurts to touch?

_____

_____

_____

_____

_____

_____

What are your thoughts/plans for dealing with any re-maining emotions or cancer personality traits that are still strong?

_____

_____

_____

_____

_____

_____

_____

CHAPTER VII

The Diagnosis: My Invitation to a New Life

On July 4, 2001 I found a lump under my left arm. I discovered it doing my usual soaping in the shower. Literally, it was not there one day but was there the next. The mammogram and the ultrasound did not show anything in my breasts, but my doctor still thought I should have the lump biopsied. I booked an appointment with an oncology surgeon. She did not think it was anything to worry about, either. On Friday, the 13th of July, I had it biopsied. (No kidding, these are the real dates.) The oncology surgeon came into the recovery room while I was still groggy from the anesthesia and baldly announced: "I'm sorry, it's cancer."

I was shell-shocked. I looked around me in the surgical recovery room to see who the surgeon was talking to. But, oh yes, she was looking at me, a woman who had done so much to eat healthy, a woman who took so many vitamins, a woman who had cleaned up so much of her physical environment.

The surgeon kept talking. I heard her somewhere out there in the fog. I only focused in on her again when I heard: "Because it's in your lymphatic system, it's at least Stage 2. This means we have to act quickly. We will book you for a double mastectomy next Tuesday, and then you will need to do chemotherapy and radiation."

How could this be? Oh no, no, no. They must have mixed up my biopsy with someone else's. Some other poor woman was walking around who had cancer. But not me. It couldn't be me, it just couldn't. I had spent the previous nine years battling a dysfunctional immune system and I thought I was winning that battle. I had done so much to clean up my diet and environment; how could this be true?

My disbelief grabbed hold of me. It was as if time stopped. Looking back, it felt like a true "out of body" experience. All I could think of was that I was going to die. The fear was immense. How could I have cancer when I was doing everything right? As soon as I asked that question, I realized something must be very wrong with my life, with my soul, with my mind—with me. Something—maybe many things—were out of balance, out of control. Thinking back, I came to the conclusion that perhaps this *was* connected to the previous nine years. Remember, the doctors said they couldn't fix my problem, that all they could do was to treat the symptoms. They could not make the disease itself go away.

"I'm sorry, it's cancer"

I went home and spent hours crying and mourning, because I was sure I was going to die. My husband came out at 2:30 a.m. and tried to help me snap out of my pity party by saying to me, "You are keeping me awake. You are the first person to tell everybody else to do their research and here you are just letting the doctor tell you what to do!" It stopped the pity party for a moment, but then I thought, "Hey, what does *he* know? *He* hasn't just been given a death sentence!" I went back to the pity party.

Then I heard God for the second time in my life. A voice said, "Do not worry." Again, my first thought was that someone had broken into the house. Then I realized that, just like the first time, it was a voice inside me. It filled the room, but it was resonating inside me. Again, I could not tell you if it was a male or female voice, but it was a voice and I knew it was God. "I love you and I will not let anything bad happen to you; you must have faith in Me." It was exactly the same wording as the first time. And I "got" it. I had an epiphany. The voice reminded me that, even if the worst happened and I died, I would be going to a better place. I believe in Heaven, you see. So I knew right then that, no matter what, I was going to be just fine. I reasoned that if I died I would be going to God and if I lived I would have things that could help others.

All of a sudden, the fear was gone and I felt instead a sense of purpose and energy. I realized I had the whole weekend in which to study the doctor's recommendations for surgery, chemo, and radiation. So I turned on the computer and got to work. There was not a great deal out there on the internet in 2001, but the information I found was very helpful. By the end of the weekend, I did not know exactly what I was going to do, but I knew what I was **not** going to do.

I'm a firm believer in "knowledge is power." Here are some things my research turned up that weekend:

On cancer—

- **By the time a tumor shows up, it has usually been growing in the body for at least two years, and perhaps as much as 10 years.** Thus, unless it is a very aggressive cancer, the patient has the time to make an informed decision. Too many times, oncologists and surgeons play on your fears and schedule you for their services the next day or the next week. By then, they have you as a patient, a customer. Truth is, you **do** have time to ask questions, look at the cancer statistics, and find out—among other things—why the cancer survival rates are so poor and why the "war on cancer" was declared a failure after 40 years.[4]

- **Cancer cells are smart.** Like weeds in the garden, they know when you are trying to kill them, and they build immunities and resistance to chemo and radiation. I am sure you have heard at least one story of someone going

---

4 Kolata G. Forty Years War-Pledged to Find and Answer, but Advances Elusive in the Drive to Cure Cancer. *New York Times*. April 24, 2009

through cancer treatment to whom the doctors have said, "I am sorry, we have tried everything, and there is nothing left to offer."

- **Regular cells have a birth, a life cycle, and a death.**
Cancer cells have only a birth; then they live until the person dies. I believe that this is the only way in which cancer is stupid. If it were really an intelligent animal, it would keep the host alive as so many infections do.

- **Something everyone should know: cancer craves sugar.**
This statement is proven during PET/CT Scans where, when they inject the patient with radioactive sugar, the resulting films show lit up areas where the sugar has been absorbed by the cancer.

Cancer also loves stress, negative emotions, fear, and anger—probably because they weaken the immune system, which makes the cancer stronger. There are MRIs that show the immune system part of the brain shutting down with negative words and emotions, while the part of the brain that creates stress hormones—the ones that feed cancer—lights up.

- **The immune system cannot see cancer.**
Cancer cells often camouflage themselves to look like something familiar and harmless. Cancer cells can secrete proteins and create biofilms[5] to cloak themselves from the immune system's defenses.

- **If cancer is not growing, it is dying.**
This is very important! Its whole purpose is to thrive and grow, so when a cancer remains the same, even if it does not get smaller, that is a powerful sign. Too many people get discouraged if their tests show that the cancer is the same. But what it really means is that you have regained the upper hand in your cancer dance.

---

5 *Merriam Webster Dictionary* defines *biofilm* as "a thin usually resistant layer of microorganisms (as bacteria) that form on and coat various surfaces."

On surgery—

- **Surgery is an assault upon the body.**

  Anything invasive is just that—you are invading the body. The same holds true here. Surgery causes emotional and physical stress, and the anesthesia is toxic.

- **It is a medical fact that surgery stimulates cancer and causes metastases**[6, 7]

  It has been proven to cause metastasis, which is when clumps of cancer cells break off from the main site and spread elsewhere in the body.

- **When a tumor is removed, regular Circulating Tumor Cells are replaced with Circulating Stem Cells.**

  According to Dr. Max Wicha, the reason breast cancer and other malignancies often return aggressively after treatment is that when tumor cells die under assault from chemotherapy and radiation, they give off substances that can reactivate a special set of master cells known as cancer stem cells. The Wicha laboratory, a leader in Cancer Stem Cell (CSC) biology has found has found that inflammatory molecules secreted by dying tumor cells can hook up with the stem cells and cause them, in effect, to come out of hibernation. Conventional medicine currently has no way to treat cancer stem cells. This is the main reason that metastatic cancer kills.

- **Surgery weakens the body and the immune system.**[8]

  Anything that weakens the immune system strengthens the cancer. No matter what school of medicine you subscribe to, all agree that cancer is first and foremost a failure of the immune system.

---

6 http://www.health-science-spirit.com/Krokowski.pdf (1979)

7 http://www.mdpi.com/2072-6694/2/2/305/pdf (March 2010)

8 http://www.breastcancer.org/tips/immune/cancer/surgery

On both conventional chemotherapy and radiation—

Each one:

- Kills the P53 tumor-suppressor gene, the very gene you need to fight cancer.
- Distorts the DNA of your healthy cells, making them pre-cancerous.
- Weakens the immune system.
- Damages vital body organs.
- Promotes tumor growth and spread.[9]
- Causes the cancer to build immunities against it.
- Has many violent side-effects on other organs, severely impacting quality-of-life.

When I started my research the Friday of my biopsy and initial diagnosis, I was merely trying to find out what I was facing, what I was about to go through. I didn't have any up-close and personal experience with cancer, other than seeing other people walk around bald, sick, and dying.

What I learned that weekend told me how damaging the surgeon's solution was going to be. Everything about her protocol would make the cancer stronger. It didn't seem like a very smart thing to do and went against everything I had learned in the last nine years, which was: repair your body. By the end of the weekend, I firmly believed that my body couldn't handle a brutal regimen of surgery, radiation, and chemo. And my mind couldn't imagine being bald and boobless and still seeing myself as a powerful woman and a confident sexual being. Sunday morning, I remember thinking I would rather die with all my body parts intact. I concluded I should die with dignity and as much quality-of-life as I could manage.

Monday morning was my pre-op appointment. I was confident that no matter what happened I would be fine. I didn't know yet what

---

9 http://cancerres.aacrjournals.org/content/early/2011/09/28/0008-5472. CAN-11-0627.full.pdf

I was going to do, but I knew what I was *not* going to do, and I was definitely equipped with the facts to support that decision. The conversation went something like this:

ME: Doctor, is it true that conventional therapy:
- Kills the P53 tumor-suppressor gene;
- Weakens the immune system and vital body organs;
- Distorts the DNA of your healthy cells, making them pre-cancerous;
- Strengthens cancer and causes metastases;
- Causes cancer to build immunities against the chemo and radiation?

DOCTOR: Yes, that is all true.

ME: Why would I want to do that?

DOCTOR: Because it is all we can offer.

ME: I cannot believe it is all that is out there for me. I'm going to look around.

DOCTOR: If you don't do the mastectomy, chemo and radiation that we have planned for you, you will probably die.

ME: God is the only one who knows when I am going to die; you just have an opinion.

However, my confidence was soon shaken.

The next week, additional scans in Houston showed lesions in my brain and lungs. They were now saying, "Advanced-Stage Metastatic Breast Cancer." I knew enough at this point not to let him give me a stage number, because that would have a negative impact on my mind and its relationship to the body.

My oncologist said to "get my affairs in order," that I probably wouldn't see another birthday—just five months away—no matter what I did. In fact, he said it would be more like three months at the outside. His recommendations were pretty much a carbon copy of the surgeon's; he still strongly recommended a double mastectomy, chemo,

and radiation. I refused again. He said I must start the process immediately, starting with a double mastectomy. I told him I would make
him a deal: he could cut off his body parts first and tell me what he felt
about it. I would then make up my mind. He then yelled at me that I
was going to die. I said very loudly back to him, "God is the only one
who knows when I am going to die; everyone else just has an opinion,
including you!" By now, I was really beginning to feel the power in
those words.

Next I told him he was fired. He said, "You cannot fire me."

The way I figured it was that by choosing him as my oncologist, I
had hired him; therefore, I most certainly could fire him. Note: I am
not saying that you should disrespect your physician. But I felt very
strongly that his opinion would color our relationship—and my outcome—in a very negative way from that point on.

I called my HMO health plan and told them to replace him with
a compassionate, open-minded doctor who could be a member on my
team. After some argument, they did. They found a woman in the
HMO who didn't ridicule vitamins and realized that I didn't need anyone yelling at me that I was going to die.

Everywhere I turned, the peer pressure was almost overwhelming.
Everybody I knew was shocked and horrified that I was not going to go
straight into conventional therapy. The research that I had done helped
tremendously. I was able to point out to them what the dangers were
with conventional therapy and the reason why I was not going to do
that. But the herd mentality was strong. Like sheep, we Americans have
been subjected to endless messages over the years to do as the doctor
says, no questions asked. People gave me a sad shake-of-the-head and
directed a sympathetic expression my way as they silently consigned
me to the grave. Eventually they left me alone and waited for me to die.

However, I did get support for my approach from my parents and
a few old friends. They all had been part of my healing opportunities
over the years and had seen the successes that I had. They also knew
that, based on my funky immune system, the traditional approach

would most likely kill me. Also, nobody wants to see their loved ones go through the life/death struggle that conventional medicine offers.

There were a few people who could not resist putting pressure on me to take the traditional approach. To them, I finally said: "If I do what you want me to do and I die, I am going to be really pissed off and I'm going to come back and haunt you! But if I do what I wanted to do and I die, well, that was my choice."

I believe it is our life and death and, therefore, it should be our choice as much as possible.

I went for a second opinion from an oncologist at the Cancer Therapy and Research Center at the University of Texas Health Science Center in San Antonio. What a change! He was so charming and handsome that everyone called him "Doc Hollywood." He managed to take my mind off cancer for, oh, about a whopping 30 seconds. But he was never more beautiful to me than when he took the time to go through my box of records from the previous nine years, asking questions the entire time, and then saying, "I believe conventional therapy would kill you faster and much more unpleasantly than just letting the cancer do it."

He did have one conventional therapy that he recommended: hormonal therapy in the form of two estrogen blockers. He explained that, because I was estrogen/progesterone positive (ER+/PR+), estrogen was feeding the cancer. In fact, about 80 percent of breast cancers are "estrogen positive." So the estrogen blocker would help starve the cancer. The fun part about estrogen blockers was that it would put me into menopause immediately. *Do not pass GO, do not collect $200; go directly to MENOPAUSE!*

He told me about Zolodex injections in the belly. They actually shut down the ovaries' production of estrogen. You could do them once/month or one/three months. Because the needle is huge, the injections are very uncomfortable; I chose the one shot every three months.

The other hormone blocker was Femara, an aromatase inhibitor medication. Interesting phenomenon here: When the ovaries stop creating estrogen (which they would do with the Zolodex), the adrenals step in and create an estrogen-like substance called aromatase.

His other treatment recommendation? Basically, just let the cancer take me over time and enjoy a better quality of life than I would have with surgery, radiation, and chemo.

He lifted a huge weight off my shoulders. At the time I was diagnosed, there were very few people to talk to about their experiences with cancer who had not done the one-size-fits-all conventional approach. There were not many survivor stories and very few statistics. It was automatically assumed by everyone from my doctors and my family down to the check-out lady at the grocery store that I would be doing conventional therapy. The pressure was fierce and passionate. Alternative Medicine was regarded as something not worthwhile.

The good news, after this second opinion, was that I would not have to try to fight cancer while dealing with all of the side-effects of conventional therapy. The bad news was that, whatever I chose to do, I would be doing it against the mainstream of medical experience and knowledge, and what was considered conventional wisdom by most people.

CHAPTER VIII

Take Control

THINGS I LEARNED DURING MY JOURNEY

*Y*ou have to peel the "cancer" off your face and pull it out of your ears and strip it off your body so that you can see again, think again, move again. This allows you to take control of your life and destiny, which is as it should be.

You need to be the one to make the decision of what therapy you are going to do—not the doctor, not your spouse, not your family or friends. Remember, if you accept someone else's direction and die, you'll have died through letting others choose for you. They will still be alive, but you will be very dead.

I have spoken to many other cancer patients since 2001, and they all had similar feelings about their reaction to the diagnosis:

- **You feel as if you are blinded.**
  You feel blinded by the panic and fear; it is as if your eyes are covered over with the word CANCER and you cannot see around it.

- **You feel as if you have gone deaf.**
  It is as if your ears are blocked by the words I AM GOING TO DIE, and you cannot hear anything else.

- **You become a "deer in the headlights," as if you are watching a speeding car coming straight towards you, and you cannot move.**

Your mind and body feel frozen in place. Your heart is beating so fast, and you are shaking inside, and all the stories and "snapshots in time" of people you have known who have been in your situation are running through your mind—most of them bad. You are in a panic to do something NOW, to rip out this deadly thing that has grown inside you, but you don't know which way to turn.

- **You adopt the sheep method.**

Most people's first impulse—mine, too—is to turn to the doctor and say, "What can I do? What are my options?" What we are basically saying is, "Save me. Tell me what to do. I will do whatever you say." This is the sheep mentality where we follow along blindly. The best illustration about the dangers in this behavior that I have ever come across was expressed in the following news article from July 8, 2005[10]:

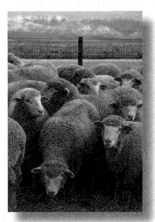

450 sheep leapt to their deaths in the Turkish village of Gevas. The chain reaction started when one sheep went over the cliff, enticing nearly fifteen hundred others to follow. According to the Aksam newspaper, by the time the 450 had died, the pile of sheep carcasses at the bottom of the cliff had apparently grown large enough to cushion the fall somewhat, resulting in the saving of the other 1050.

When I was young, and I wanted to follow the current fashions, my mother used to say, "If everyone stuck beans up their nose, would you?" Well, the answer is "yes" for most people. How many times have we heard "go with the flow," or "stick with the status quo," or "there is safety in numbers." We figure if most people are doing something, that thing must be the best thing to do. Not true. Let me give you an example.

---

10 https://en.wikinews.org/wiki/450_sheep_leap_to_their_deaths_in_Turkey

Going with the flow in the computer industry

As a software consultant in the computer industry, I worked for DEC. We did things slightly different than IBM, and we were the second largest computer corporation in the world, right behind IBM. Our systems and software were hands-down better than IBM. The only reason we were second was because we weren't IBM. We didn't advertise, so we were not a household name. We hadn't been around as long as IBM, either, so we were the new kid on the block. We were different, not the norm. When people had computer needs, they went first to IBM. The belief was "IBM is the biggest, and most businesses use them, so they must be the best." There you have it: sheep blindly following other sheep.

Going with the flow in your medical treatment

You may think, "Yes, but computers are not about life and death. Doctors are not IBM salesmen; they have been through extensive schooling. And I would go to someone very experienced, someone who had been practicing medicine for years."

Actually, even with my nine years of experience with the fallibility of doctors fresh in my mind, those were my initial thoughts. I turned to my surgeon, who had just given me the diagnosis, and said, "What can I do? What are my options?" Remember that I was told the recommendation, since the tumor was not readily visible and that it was at least Stage II, would be a double mastectomy instead of a single mastectomy, followed by chemo and radiation. Quietly, some oncologists used to tell you that if they or their spouse got cancer, they would never agree to undergo the standard chemo regimen they perform every day on patients like you and me. Yet at the office, the sheep fall in line and do as they are told because there is safety in numbers—a doctor probably won't get sued if he or she does what everyone else is doing. And it's profitable for the doctors.

The surgeon had told me she could fit me in the following Tuesday for the operation. And I had agreed. The Deer-in-the-Headlights thing was happening to me.

So, how did I peel off the "cancer" and take control? I did it by getting empowered through knowledge. Today, it is easy to confuse knowledge with information with marketing. Those with something to sell pay to get their message out often so we see it again and again and these sales pitches shape our perception. We are overwhelmed with information meant to influence our decisions and how we spend our money. The kind of objective *knowledge* needed to make a major decision like, how best to treat cancer, comes from questioning, searching, and critically examining what the cancer establishment and other sources tell us. Cancer is big business and that colors the advice cancer patients often get.

> ### *The most important thing I learned during my journey is to build a solid, integrated holistic platform to place the chosen therapy for cancer and chronic disease.*

The day of your birth is the first day of the rest of your life. *Literally*. But the day of your cancer diagnosis *becomes* the first day of the rest of your life in a very realistic and personal manner. I have spoken to many cancer patients and survivors, and they all tell me how they began to live each day in a more magnified, focused, intense manner. When your "death date" is given to you by your oncologist or surgeon, it becomes very real.

News Flash: We all die—nobody gets out alive!

Whether you end up living into your 90s or whether you die tomorrow in a car accident, your diagnosis day is the first day of the rest of your life.

Which begs the questions:

- How do I want to live?
- How do I want to die?

I researched survivors. I found that most of them followed a program. By program, I mean a grouping of elements that make up a whole, coordinated approach. Well, that was good, because I had nine years of experience with a grouping of elements that make up a whole, coordinated approach: my holistic Healing Platform. I was on the right track.

After more research, I set up my **Healing Platform** for cancer.

Go back to your diagnosis. Write about the process, the tests, the diagnosis itself, and your feelings.

_____

_____

_____

_____

_____

_____

_____

_____

_____

_____

_____

_____

Write about your research, the pressures of doctors, family, friends, and how it made you feel. How did you respond? Were you able to release the pressure?

_____

_____

_____

_____

_____

_____

_____

_____

_____

_____

_____

_____

_____

_____

_____

Bring up the negative emotions so you can recognize and purge them. Get rid of the dis-ease associated with your memories of the diagnosis. If you cannot purge them just yet, make note of them to deal with later in your detox modality. What do you still need to purge?

_____

_____

_____

_____

_____

_____

_____

_____

_____

_____

_____

_____

Write about things you learned during this portion of your journey. Everything.

_____

_____

_____

_____

_____

_____

_____

_____

_____

_____

_____

_____

_____

Have you used any of it?

_____

_____

_____

_____

_____

_____

Did you find it to your advantage?

_____

_____

_____

_____

_____

_____

_____

Are you still using it?

_____

_____

_____

_____

_____

What healing modality does it fall under: Nutrition, Spirituality, Mind-Body, Detox, etc.?

_____

_____

_____

_____

_____

_____

_____

_____

Then write about the rest of your life. How do you want to live?

_____

_____

_____

_____

_____

_____

How do you want to die?

_____

_____

_____

_____

_____

_____

NOW, let's create your Healing Platform!

CHAPTER IX

What Is a Healing Platform, And Why Is It Important?

*M*ost doctors and patients approach illness from a strictly physical point of view. What are the physical symptoms? What pill, operation, action, or therapy can make the *symptoms* go away? We in Western society have been trained to go to the doctor at the first sign of illness so that the doctor can "fix" the symptoms with traditional western medicine, which typically employs pharmaceutical products and a scalpel. We have also been taught to make full use of vaccines against illness as a preventative measure. Yet most of these approaches have toxic side-effects that damage the immune system and vital body organs. These unnatural interventions can also have emotionally and psychologically damaging effects on us.

My approach to cancer was to dig down deep and find the reasons the cancer got strong enough to unbalance my immune system and take over my body. I wanted to find the causes of the dis-ease, the dysfunctions in my life that showed up in my body. I believe that cancer and the tumors, etc., are symptoms of the disease, and that your body is trying to tell you something is out of balance and needs to be adjusted: either added to, taken away from, or just tweaked.

The symptoms are the messengers. You've heard that old saying, "Don't shoot the messenger?" It's true; you should listen to the messenger and find the value in the message itself. Getting a diagnosis of a tumor is a bit like having the "check engine" light come on the car dash. Do you beat the dash with a hammer until the light goes out? No. You take it to the shop and find out what the problem is. That's what we need to do with a tumor. Let's first find out why we have a problem before we decide how to address it.

I took my existing healing platform and reexamined it. In each instance, I searched my life, mind, body, and soul for "dis-ease." What didn't feel right? What did I need to change or take out? What did I need to add?

I discovered that I needed to ramp up my focus on all of them but especially detox, immune boosting, spirituality, and mind/body.

My first attempt at the Healing Platform for cancer consisted of the following modalities:

- spirituality
- mind/body
- immunity
- nourishment/nutrition
- detox
- lifestyle

For the next year, I employed this holistic approach with the only other cancer therapy being the Zolodex® and Femara®. However, in July of 2002, exactly one year after my diagnosis, I found more swollen lymph nodes. I knew the cancer was on the move again and that I needed to add a formal medical cancer therapy to my holistic platform.

Another important thing I learned during my journey is to "Choose wisely, Grasshopper"

What I had been doing held it off for a year and gave me another year of life, which was already much longer than the doctors had given me. But it was not enough. It is important that you stay positive about your chosen therapy, but do not close your eyes and refuse to see the elephant in the room. If you find that what you are doing is not working exactly as you think it should, examine it carefully, get other opinions, do more research, and consider tweaking the therapy or changing it.

I knew that I had to tweak my healing platform. I knew I had to add something very powerful, a therapy that would be hard on the cancer and yet still be easy on me, my body, and my immune system. I knew I needed a targeted cancer therapy aspect to my platform.

Now my healing platform looked like this:

- spirituality
- mind/body
- immunity
- nourishment/nutrition
- detox
- lifestyle
- **targeted cancer therapy**

When I examined the emotions and thoughts behind each modality, I realized that they had prioritized themselves and that they inspired different feelings in me. The familiarity of the order and the feelings reminded me of an old meditation tape that dealt with the chakras, the colors associated with them, the "spinning" of them, and the feelings they invoked.

It was like fitting puzzle pieces together into the finished whole: The Healing Platform™ followed the chakras and encompassed the whole being, the entire body/mind/soul of the person:

- **Spirituality**
- **Mind/Body**
- **Immunity**
- **Nourishment**
- **Detox**
- **Lifestyle**
- **Targeted Therapy of Choice**

The Healing Platform

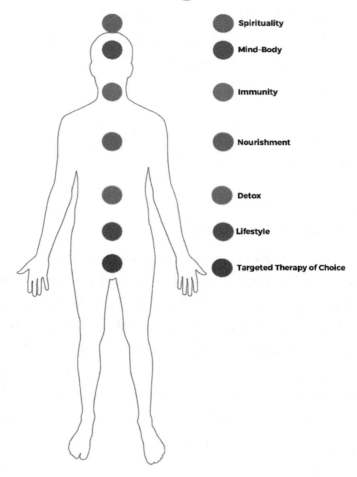

Spirituality

Mind-Body

Immunity

Nourishment

Detox

Lifestyle

Targeted Therapy of Choice

© Best Answer For Cancer Foundation

But why the chakras, you may be asking. Why not just a color-coded table, if I like color?

We are trained that tables and charts help make order out of chaos, so I wanted to manage my particular health "chaos" with some sort of pictorial chart. When I thought about the chakras, it made sense to me that, if I believed my cancer treatment needed to embody all aspects of mind, body, soul, and spirit, then the aspects of the chakras would fit and give me an age-old connectivity between the energy aspects of mind, body, soul, and spirit. Here is what I found from the Brofman

Foundation for the Advancement of Healing that explained the chakras in part:

> The chakras are described as being aligned in an ascending column from the base of the spine to the top of the head. In New Age practices, each chakra is often associated with a certain color. In various traditions chakras are associated with multiple physiological functions, an aspect of consciousness, a classical element, and other distinguishing characteristics.
>
> The chakras are thought to vitalize the physical body and to be associated with interactions of a physical, emotional and mental nature. The function of the chakras is to spin and draw in this energy to keep the spiritual, mental, emotional and physical health of the body in balance. They are said by some to reflect how the unified consciousness of humanity (the immortal human being or the soul), is divided to manage different aspects of earthly life (body/instinct/vital energy/deeper emotions/communication/having an overview of life/contact to God). The chakras are placed at differing levels of spiritual subtlety, with Sahasrara at the top being concerned with pure consciousness, and Muladhara at the bottom being concerned with matter, which is seen simply as condensed or gross consciousness.

Understanding the chakras allows you to understand the relationship between your consciousness and your body, and to thus see your body as a map of your consciousness.

I then set about fleshing out my platform with therapies, products, procedures, etc., that I felt would solve the dis-ease in my life. These things have changed over the years, as my life has changed and my knowledge has grown. The platform has given me the ability to flex, to address changes in my life as I go along.

Patients ask me to give them concrete therapies, products, and procedures for this platform. That I will not do, as the platform must be unique to the individual. This individuality is also the reason I don't believe there is *a* cure for cancer. I think cancer is the result of a combination of factors that makes up the perfect storm and results in cancer.

The storm is your particular stew of personal factors, genetics, environmental toxins, diet, lifestyle: all the issues that make up your "dis-ease." I believe cancer is the true Yuppie disease—unique to the individual. Therefore, what works for one person will not necessarily work for another person with the same type of cancer. This book is your opportunity to explore yourself and build your own cure.

There are many choices for each modality in the healing platform; I'll present my philosophy and thoughts on each one as well as some choices, but the actual platform needs to be tailored to the individual and his or her lifestyle.

Another reason not to fill in the blanks for you is that I am a firm believer in each person taking ownership of their illness, doing their own research, and making their own decisions. It is the sense of empowerment and ownership that I am wishing for you and trying to give you. Until and unless you are making your own decisions about your treatment, you will not be a contributor to the outcome.

Also keep in mind that most options are not—and probably should not—be static. The body can get used to something and even build a sort of immunity against it. If we are talking specifically about cancer, it does indeed build immunities to things. Changing things around is also good for you; it gives you something new to experience and adds a bit of variety to your life.

Your Mission

We now need to set up your Healing Platform chart and start filling it in. You can make your own chart fairly easily. Start with a ruled pad of paper. You can always transfer your notes to a more formal chart later.

As we go through the modalities in the next seven chapters, list each modality (i.e., Spirituality, Mind/Body, etc.) along with your chosen therapies, your notes, and your decisions. Add the items from your previous exercises that you may have used for any prior illnesses. Then in a separate column list your anticipated start date and stop date for each therapy/item within the modality. Remember not to have patterns for the stop/start that cancer can learn. For instance, do one supplement therapy for 5 weeks, the next for 3, the following one for 6, etc.

Some tips: With supplements, I actually transferred start and stop dates to a regular calendar, so that I had a visual of what was supposed to happen then. I would set alarms on my computer to alert me a day or so in advance that I had a switch coming up. Even with a specific diet, I switched foods I was eating all the time, being careful not to eat the same foods in any sort of pattern. It kept things interesting for me, too!

Make some notes below about items you don't want to forget, or issues you know of right now that you want to make sure you address. Once you have done that, and you have your healing platform outline in front of you...

Let's get started!

THINGS WE MUST NOT FORGET:

_____

_____

_____

_____

_____

_____

_____

_____

_____

_____

_____

_____

_____

_____

_____

_____

_____

_____

_____

_____

_____

_____

_____

_____

_____

CHAPTER X

Spirituality

*U*sually, when I bring up God or spirituality, people have one of two reactions: they proudly proclaim their religious beliefs, or they start shutting down. When I hear other people talk about the role of God or spirit in healing, they usually put it last, almost as if they are embarrassed by it. But what I found when I started researching the role of spirituality in medicine was that it had a great basis in healing.

The database on the National Institutes of Health's library website Pubmed.com has 5,347 studies listed for "spirituality and health," and 1,287 studies for spirituality and cancer.

One study was conducted from 1992 to 2012 of 74,534 women on the association of attendance at religious services and mortality. The conclusion was: "Frequent attendance at religious services was associated with significantly lower risk of all-cause, cardiovascular, and cancer mortality among women. Religion and spirituality may be an underappreciated resource that physicians could explore with their patients, as appropriate."[11]

As reported in *Clinical Journal of Oncology Nurses* in an article entitled *Assessment and Implementation of Spirituality and Religiosity in*

---

11 Li S, Stampfer MJ et all. Association of Religious Service Attendance With Mortality Among Women. *JAMA Intern Med.* 2016 June 1;176(6):777-85. Doi 10.1001/jamainternmed.2016.1615.

Cancer Survival,[12] patients with cancer who engage in activities that promote a positive spiritual well-being have been described as having a greater quality of life, making more aggressive care choices to extend life, and reporting satisfaction with care provided. Conversely, patients who do not receive adequate spiritual care become distressed, leading to poorer outcomes such as increased pain, feelings of isolation, hopelessness, and anger.

If you search PubMed for spirituality and cancer, it turns out the studies are actually talking more about how spirituality adds to the quality of life, but not how spirituality adds to survival. It is as if spirituality has been relegated to the back burner in conventional medicine. Spirituality is a nice icing on the cake, but nothing more. I sometimes call spirituality the "purple" side of cancer. It's awkward for doctors to even get near it because they don't want to talk "religion" with patients. And there is no business model for making money in the doctor's office when dealing with spirituality.

However, I think it is also a grave disservice to the healing power that is available through the tools in this realm. I have been handed three clearly-defined and definite death sentences thus far, and I am still alive. Why is that, you may ask? Was it the choices I made in medical therapies? That most likely had something to do with it. However, you will never convince me that God did not have *a lot* to do with it. It is my belief that God blessed my broken body with extra time, and that I am here for a specific purpose.

I have an advantage over most people in that I heard God's voice twice. I have never heard it since the time I was diagnosed with end-stage cancer, and there have been times that I began to doubt. But then I remembered. These days, I do not doubt. I just have faith. For those who have not had a personal experience with God, I can offer mine as something to hold on to.

---

12 Richardson P. Assessment and Implementation of Spirituality and Religiosity in Cancer Survival. CJON 2012, 16(4), E150-E155 DOI: 10.1188/12.CJON.E150-E155

People have told me that they wait for God to show them the path, to tell them what to do. I have personally never done that. I live by the "God helps those who help themselves" system. I also think this joke is apropos:

> The flood waters are rising. The sheriff sends a truck, then a boat, then a helicopter, but the man won't leave, saying, "God will save me." When he gets to heaven he says, "God, where were you?" and God says, "What do you mean: I sent a truck, a boat, and a helicopter!"

If you don't already have a relationship with God, a Supreme Energy Source, a Higher Power, or a spiritual belief system, I sincerely suggest you should consider finding one, or at least open yourself up to the possibility. It is important to believe that there is something bigger and more powerful than you that is aiding in your healing. I found it invaluable to be able to "give it up" to something bigger when the going got tough. It was also nice that, when the doctor told me in 2001 that I was going to die very soon, I was able to say with quiet confidence "HE is the only one who knows I am going to die; YOU just have an opinion."

One of my favorite phrases is: *"God is Large and In Charge"*

Even if you don't believe in God or the power of prayer, you have to believe in something more powerful than you or the cancer. Something more than you can touch, see, or taste, because this experience is too tough to go through without something to hold on to. Some being that inspires awe by its very nature. Some being that you can give it all up to. Some being that can bear the burden for you when you get overwhelmed.

Spirituality is often understood to be less dogmatic than religion. Whereas religions often have one prescribed path to God, spirituality can see many paths to God or a Higher Power. Religion is usually practiced in a formal house of worship at set times; spirituality is something you can practice on the beach 24/7; it does not have to be associated with a particular day or hour. To me, spirituality has always referred to my connection with a Higher Power, or God.

How does prayer fit in? Sometimes prayer is something individual; sometimes it is very public as in a church, synagogue, or mosque. There have been many studies on the efficacy of prayer, beginning as early as Francis Galton's 1872 study.

Perhaps the two most powerful studies are explained below in an article on the power of prayer in healing by Vijai P. Sharma, Ph.D.

Studies Find That Prayer Can Help the Sick[13]
Vijai P. Sharma, Ph.D

A study on prayer fascinated me and I want to share it with you.

This study was conducted by Dr. Randolph Byrd, a heart specialist at the San Francisco General Hospital. This is how it went.

Dr. Byrd took four hundred patients who were admitted to the Hospital's Cardiac Intensive-Care Unit. He divided them in to two groups: one group received regular medical care of the hospital, called the "control group"; the second group received not only regular medical care but also prayers, called the "prayer group."

To eliminate any selection bias, he let the computer randomly assign patients to one of the two groups. People who met to pray for the prayer group were given just the names of the patients and very preliminary information on their medical condition. All patients, belonging to either of the groups, signed a consent form, informing them of the possibility that they might or might not get prayed for. So none of the patients knew whether he or she actually got prayed for and at the same time, every one stood an equal chance.

Needless to say that all patients, their friends and relatives were free to pray on their own if they wanted to. No suggestion was made about self initiated prayers one way or the other.

13 http://www.mindpub.com/art031.htm. Reprinted with permission.

The point I am making is that these being such large groups, all chance factors would equal out to make a strict comparison between the prayer group and the control group. This enabled the researchers to objectively study the effect of the additional prayers that were organized by the hospital.

Furthermore, neither the staff, nor the patient knew who was being prayed for. This is really important in a scientific study because if the patients know or find out about such differences, then, arguably, they may improve or get worse due to the placebo effect.

For instance, the one who is prayed for, may get an additional psychological booster and the other who knows he is not being prayed, may feel deprived of something that may have a potential for improvement.

By the same token, it is important that the treatment staff not know which patient is participating in which group. Understandably, if a member of the treatment team knows about the composition of the groups, they may give certain patients preferential treatment, give them more attention, or pass" on, unintentionally, their hope and enthusiasm to the patient. All told, as concerns the standards of unbiased and objective study, it met all the requirements.

Now for the results of the study.

Dr. Byrd found that the prayed for group did much better than the group that was not prayed for. Several benefits were noted for the group that was prayed for, they were much less likely to develop congestive heart failure and pulmonary edema in which the lungs fill with fluid; they were five times less likely to require antibiotics; fewer needed to be put on ventilators and receive artificial respiration; fewer developed pneumonia or had cardiac arrests. All the benefits mentioned above were statistically significant.

Studies following respectable scientific standards have also been conducted comparing the effectiveness of the various types of prayer. One such study comes from the Spindrift Foundation in Salem, Oregon, which specializes in prayer studies.

For the purpose of this study, prayers are classified in two types; the "directed prayer" and the "undirected prayer." Let us see how they define the two types.

A directed prayer has a specific wish and a specific outcome in mind.

Nondirected prayer is just the consciousness of who is being prayed for. The prayer is simply for the best potential of the individual to manifest or the best outcome to happen for that person. So nondirected prayer is "thy will be done" type of prayer.

This study was also done on the germination of seeds. The seeds that were prayed for always germinated more than the seeds that were not prayed for, and the seeds that received nondirected prayers germinated more than the ones that received directed prayers.

Spindrift Foundation concluded that both types of prayers were beneficial, but the non-directed prayers were three to four times more effective.

My personal bias, which is not based on any scientific study, is that a prayer for changing oneself into a better person is more desirable than the prayers for some material benefits. I am aware that my bias may have been determined by the fact that I am a psychologist and I am in the business of personal change.

After reading about the Spindrift Foundation Study concluding that non-directed prayer was three to four times more effective, all of my prayers were for my highest good instead of specific healing of the cancer. I also enlisted the aid of a local church. I was on the Prayer List and I attended the weekly healing service where I received "laying on of hands" as well as group prayer.

I had no specific time for prayer other than first thing in the morning and last thing at night. In the morning, I followed prayer with counting my blessings and in the evening I preceded prayer with counting my blessings. Prayer was always the way I began and ended the day.

Meditation

I found a wonderful blog by John Paul Fanton on the website Healthy Fellow on meditation. http://www.healthyfellow.com/385/meditation-and-cancer/. The following is reprinted with his permission.

> A study reported in 2009 done at *St. Mary's College* in Fukuoka, Japan, examined the effects of a "mindfulness-based meditation therapy" on the mental health of 28 cancer patients. All the participants were receiving conventional chemotherapy and radiation treatment during the course of the trial. The meditative therapy involved two sessions. In the first, an instructor taught the patients the technique which involved breathing exercises, meditation and yoga movements. The patients then practiced these exercises at home with the assistance of a meditative CD. Measures of anxiety, depression and "spiritual wellbeing" were taken pre- and post-treatment. Anxiety and depression scores dropped by about 30% in the meditators.[14]
>
> But these results provide only a partial picture of the apparent capabilities of mindfulness:
>
> - A study on women with early stage breast cancer from the August 2008 issue of the *Brain Behavior and Immunology* found that "mindfulness based stress reduction" (MBSR) improved coping ability, immune function (Natural killer cell activity) and quality of life. A reduction in cortisol levels (a stress hormone) was also detected.[15]
> - A trial from November, 2007, discovered that a mindfulness program could decrease blood pressure, improve immune function, sleep quality and lower stress in a group of men and women with

---

14 Ando M, Morita T et al. The Efficacy of Mindfulness-Based Meditation Therapy on Anxiety, Depression, and Spirituality in Japanese Patients with Cancer. *Journal of Palliative Medicine*. December 2009, 12(12): 1091-1094. doi:10.1089/jpm.2009.0143.

15 Witek-Janusek L, Albuquerque K et al. Effect of Mindfulness Based Stress Reduction on Immune Function, Quality of Life and Coping In Women Newly Diagnosed with Early Stage Breast Cancer. *Brain Behav Immun*. 2008 August; 22(6): 969–981.

breast and prostate cancer. The results of this investigation were still evident at a one year follow up examination.[16]

There is even some research that suggests that mindfulness can positively influence the levels of select hormones, especially *DHEA* that may affect the progression of certain hormonally-influenced cancers. This is yet another exciting mechanism by which meditation and stress management may improve outcomes in cancer survivors.[17]

Healing Touch

Healing Touch is a relaxing, nurturing energy therapy. Gentle touch assists in balancing our physical, mental, emotional, and spiritual well-being. Healing Touch works with our energy field to support our natural ability to heal.

HealingTouchInternational.com reported on the following studies on healing touch and cancer:

- A randomized clinical trial was conducted with 62 women receiving radiation treatment for gynecological and breast cancer at Barnes-Jewish Hospital in St. Louis, Missouri. Comparisons of scores before and after the six treatment sessions showed significant changes in improved quality of life and proportionately larger reductions in fatigue in the Healing Touch group than the control group. The Healing Touch group demonstrated more

---

16 Carlson L, Speca M et al. One year pre–post intervention follow-up of psychological, immune, endocrine and blood pressure outcomes of mindfulness-based stress reduction (MBSR) in breast and prostate cancer outpatients. *Brain, Behavior, and Immunity*. Volume 21, Issue 8, November 2007, Pages 1038-1049

17 Carlson L, Speca M et al. Mindfulness-based stress reduction in relation to quality of life, mood, symptoms of stress and levels of cortisol, dehydroepiandrosterone sulfate (DHEAS) and melatonin in breast and prostate cancer outpatients.*Psychoneuroendocrinology*. Volume 29, Issue 4, May 2004, Pages 448-474

pronounced improvements in their levels of depression, anxiety and anger compared to the control group.[18]

- A 2003 study measured the effects of therapeutic massage and Healing Touch on pain, nausea, fatigue and anxiety in 230 chemotherapy patients in comparison to caring presence alone or standard cancer treatment alone. There was a significant immediate (after individual treatment) and overall (at the end of the four visits) effect for both massage therapy and Healing Touch. Both Healing Touch and massage reduced blood pressure and heart rate and level of pain in comparison to presence. Healing Touch and massage reduced mood disturbance during the intervention periods, although there were no specific effects on anxiety-tension. Fatigue was less in the Healing Touch period. There were no significant immediate or overall effects on nausea with massage or Healing Touch. Participants rated both interventions highly regarding overall helpfulness and satisfaction.[19]

Reiki

Energy therapies involve using the body's energy fields to heal and maintain wellness.

Although Western medicine is focused on chemical interventions, the human body is first and foremost a bio-electrical entity. Energetic interventions have no side-effects and speak to the body's native language.

Medical school teaches doctors that the heart and the brain are electrical entities and we can measure their output with monitors. As we've seen on so many TV shows, when the brain waves go flat, the body dies. When the heart beat is irregular, it's heart attack time. Conventional medical teaching doesn't go much further than that. But it should.

18 Cook CL, Guerrerio J, Slater V. The Effect of Healing Touch on Radiation-Induced Fatigue in Women Receiving Radiation Therapy in Women with Gynecological or Breast Cancer. *Alternative Therapies in Health and Medicine.* 2004, Vol. 10, No. 3, pp. 34-40.

19 Post-White J, Kinney ME et al. Therapeutic massage and healing touch improve symptoms in cancer. *Integr Cancer Ther.* 2003 Dec;2(4):332-44.

The body is about 70 percent water with a high mineral content making it highly electrically conductive.

Dr. Fritz-Albert Popp taught us that normal living cells emit a regular stream of photons—light. He proved the existence of the bio-photon field in 1974. In his book *Biologie des Lichts (Biology of Light),* he explained to us that living cells pass information to each other via photons. In other words, they talk amongst themselves by way of light.

The body has some 60- to 100-trillion cells. They work together; they must communicate in exquisitely timed sequences. The DNA sequence contracts and expands several billion times per second, producing a photon of light with each contraction.

Dr. Reinhold Voll taught us how to tap into the flow of the body's energy. In the 1950s, he verified for Western medicine what Chinese medicine had known for centuries about the use of meridians and acupuncture points for healing. Dr. Voll created a testing device that can pass a tiny electrical current through the human body and measure the amount of resistance encountered at the acupuncture points. For example, he found that patients with lung cancer had abnormal readings on the acupuncture points referred to as lung points. Today, some integrative doctors use his testing equipment to develop homeopathic remedies that can correct the body's imbalances.

On the flip side, many people are concerned now about "electrosmog pollution" from wireless networks, cell phones, cordless phones, utility company smart meters, and other devices that use energy signals that are foreign to what the body uses for communication, including pulsing microwave radiation. Most of us are smothered with this unnatural energy and evidence is mounting that can interfere with our ability to detox, it can heat our brain, and perhaps even break our DNA.

Believers in energy medicine describe disruptions in the energy field as a cause for illness and teach that balancing energy can aid in healing. Reiki is a form of energy medicine and has been evaluated in several clinical trials for treatment of anxiety and improvement of well-being in cancer patients. Unfortunately, well designed studies that can account for the placebo effect are hard to come by—who will pay for it? Yet, although there is no scientific data that fully supports these claims, patient testimonials that support reiki are numerous.

Consider what you have just read. Do you have a Higher Power that you have enough faith in to lean on when you need to, to believe in?

_____

_____

_____

_____

God, or a Higher Power, is a very complex and personal issue for most of us. Explore your spirituality by yourself in a deep, sensitive, and introspective manner. Decide what resonates within your being as an approach to this modality. If you find negative issues during this time, make a note of them and set them aside to deal with in your detox modality.

_____

_____

_____

_____

_____

SPIRITUALITY

_____

_____

_____

_____

_____

_____

_____

_____

_____

_____

_____

_____

_____

_____

_____

_____

Once you have decided on your spiritual tools, write them down and make a note as to what your schedule is to practice them. For instance, I prayed upon waking and before sleeping as a scheduled therapy, but prayer was a spontaneous part of my therapy, also.

Other things I did in this modality: I went to my church's healing service every Wednesday morning where they practiced the Laying on of Hands (a form of physical praying touch from The Order of St. Luke's). I was also on the church's prayer chain and prayer list. I did not have start and stop dates for this modality. Spirituality, unlike some of the other therapies, does not need to be varied to fool cancer. There is no evidence that cancer can build immunities against God. ☺

_____

_____

_____

_____

_____

_____

_____

_____

_____

_____

_____

_____

_____

_____

_____

_____

_____

_____

_____

_____

_____

_____

_____

_____

_____

CHAPTER XI

Mind-Body

The power of the mind over the body is immense. Dr. Joan Borysenko, author of *The Power of the Mind to Heal,* did her doctoral thesis on the mind-body connection. She studied multiple personalities. She found in several cases people had physical manifestations that would normally have been thought impossible, such as one personality having a verifiable disease that the other personalities did not.

A study reported in 2011 in *Science Translational Medicine,* for example, cast doubt over the scientific validity of nearly all randomized, double-blind placebo controlled studies involving pharmaceuticals used on human beings. Researchers found out that many pharmaceutical drugs only work because people expect them to, not because they have any "real" chemical effect on the body.[20] Previous studies on a smaller scale have found that our thoughts can affect whether painkiller drugs work, and that a placebo (empty sugar pill) outperforms antidepressant drugs as long as the people involved in the test *think* the placebo is the drug.

According to Dr. Janet Hranicky who has made using the mind-body connection for wellness her life's work:

---

20 Bingel U, Wanigasekera V et all. The Effect of Treatment Expectation on Drug Efficacy: Imaging the Analgesic Benefit of the Opioid Remifentanil. *Sci Transl Med.* February 16, 2011: Vol. 3, Issue 70, p. 70

Your beliefs and attitudes are one of the most essential factors in getting well and staying well. It is important to understand some of the foundational concepts in quantum physics to understand that the mind/brain/behavior connection in cancer consciousness represents the invisible upstream complex and organized informational template that drives all of the other downstream regulatory biochemical and genetic mechanisms that suppress tumor growth and keep the body in a healthy balanced state. Minimizing chronic stress physiology is mandatory in balancing the health of the autonomic nervous system so that the immune system and other healing systems in the body are upregulated and not consistently suppressed. Therefore, the nature and speed of healing, including spontaneous remission, correlate strongly with a person's beliefs, attitudes, spirit, and enthusiasm for life as much, if not more, as their specific diagnosis, tumor pathology, and treatment protocol.

The power of the mind over the body is a powerful weapon for the patient to use in their cancer dance.

What I like to call the **cancer dance** is a tool in itself. Consider the word dance and its many meanings. Most, if not all of them, have positive connotations and images associated with them. Research indicates that cancer is a disease that thrives on the negatives: anger, stress, bitterness, resentment, etc. If you start putting cancer thoughts, programs, and tools in a positive light, you are in effect doing something anti-cancer. Therefore, I decided that I would not have a cancer battle; I would have a cancer dance. And I would not let the cancer lead; I would take the lead in this dance.

Powerful tools include visualization, imagery, positive affirmations, and self-hypnosis.

Visualization[21]

To imagine, conceive of, see in one's mind. One of my favorite visualizations is to combine spirituality with a cancer-expunging picture. I see God coming into my body, gathering up the cancer, sweeping it out, and taking it back to Source.

Visual Imagery[22]

Make a physical image of your goal. I learned when I read *The Secret* that it really works to have a poster board on which you post pictures, words—whatever elements work for you to envision how you want your life to be. We call these things vision boards and they project a healthy, happy, prosperous, thriving you. Look at them daily and concentrate on believing that is where you are going to be.

NOTE: You can find examples and tips on Wikipedia, Huffington Post, Pinterest, Jack Canfield.com etc to get started!

Positive Affirmations[23]

An affirmation is a form of auto-suggestion in which a statement of intention is deliberately meditated on and repeated in order to implant it in the mind. Research by leading universities in the field of cognitive and behavioral science proves the existence of so called "automatic thoughts," i.e., thoughts that come to mind involuntarily and effortlessly as an automatic response to certain stimuli. These are the thoughts that ultimately determine whether you'll fail or succeed in reaching your personal goals. Your positive affirmations will be about becoming cancer-clear.

---

21 http://www.cancerresearchuk.org/cancer-help/about-cancer/treatment/complementary-alternative/therapies/visualisation#evidence

22 http://www.cancer.org/treatment/treatmentsandsideeffects/complementaryandalternativemedicine/mindbodyandspirit/imagery

23 http://www.health-science-spirit.com/cancer8-mind.html

Use Post-it notes, cards you mail yourself, sheets of paper you hang from the ceiling in your bedroom—whatever works. To this day, I still have Post-it note affirmations all over my house.

Self-hypnosis/Meditation[24]

Self-hypnosis ("autohypnosis") is a form of hypnosis which is self-induced, and normally makes use of self-suggestion. Put yourself into a meditative trance, and tell your immune system it is strong. Tell your vital body organs they are strong and cancer-free. Tell your body it is strong and cancer-free. Tell yourself you are strong and happy and unafraid. You can teach the brain to change the physiological response of your body to certain triggers.

For example, I picked a cold place to go to when I had hot flashes— I imagined myself sitting in an inner tube, flowing down an ice cold, peaceful river. In three weeks, my brain learned that every time I felt hot, it was to use this picture of me floating down the cool, serene river and send me signals that I felt cool.

Belief[25]

Belief is the psychological state in which an individual holds a proposition or premise to be true. There is something that kept me stable that first year after my cancer diagnosis when the doctors gave me my walking papers. I think a lot of that stability had to do with my denial. I just didn't want to believe I really had cancer.

Belief is a state of mind and the mind has incredible influence over the body. Use belief to your advantage. You must KNOW that you can be healed.

---

24 http://www.cancer.gov/cancertopics/pdq/supportivecare/fever/HealthProfessional/page2

25 http://www.cancer.org/treatment/treatmentsandsideeffects/complementaryandalternativemedicine/mindbodyandspirit/faith-healing

Faith

Merriam-Webster defines faith as:

1 a: allegiance to duty or a person: loyalty *b (1)*: fidelity to one's promises *(2)*: sincerity of intentions

2 a (1): belief and trust in and loyalty to God *(2)*: belief in the traditional doctrines of a religion *b (1)*: firm belief in something for which there is no proof *(2)*: complete trust

3: something that is believed especially with strong conviction; *especially*: a system of religious beliefs *<the Protestant faith>*

In this context, we are using faith as the "firm belief in something for which there is no proof." I had faith that the outcome of the cancer would be okay no matter what. If I died that I would be going to a good place and if I lived then I would be able to help others. I had faith that it would all come out as it should be.

NuCalm®

NuCalm is a patented, FDA-approved system that balances the autonomic nervous system. The autonomic nervous system (ANS) is made up of the sympathetic (fight or flight response) and parasympathetic (relaxation response) systems. In the modern world, we tend to be stressed all the time.

We eat on the run. We multi-task. We worry about jobs, finances, family, and world events. I saw a phrase recently in the newspaper that said America is "an anxiety nation." I think that says it pretty well. When we are stressed, the sympathetic side of our nervous system dominates. That means all systems are go to run away from the tiger, and things like digestion are put on the back burner. But in today's world, "the tiger" is that post-lunch meeting about a difficult project that keeps us from absorbing the nutrients in our lunch.

Relaxation is hard to come by. NaturalHealth360.com reports that, "The ANS has been studied by some researchers and was found to be out of balance in cancer patients, both after people get cancer and, more importantly, before their diagnosis." This system uses head-phones and neuroacoustic audio recordings that relax the brain, an eye mask to remove visual stimulation, a cream with gaba, and microcur-rent patches.

In Closing...

Meditation, visualization, self-hypnosis, positive thoughts, and affir-mations are all very powerful tools. I was part of a clinical trial on self-hypnosis for hot flashes for breast cancer patients. I not only got rid of the hot flashes (brought on by the cancer therapies Zolodex and Femara I used to shut down my ovaries' estrogen production), I used the same techniques to tell my body that the cancer was gone.

Research these different aspects and decide on your personal approach. I did them all, and I created a place in the house that was my Safe Place and I had a Quiet Time every morning, afternoon, and evening when I would employ my chosen techniques. Use the space below to list the tools that initially appeal to you.

_____

_____

_____

_____

_____

_____

_____

_____

_____

MIND.BODY

Take your time with this modality and really explore and research the mind-body connection until you are both awed and convinced of the power of the mind over the body. I had a practice that I developed wherein I would not let anyone's words past a virtual "barrier" in between my ears. The words could go into my ears where I would hold them until I examined their validity. If they were just someone's opinion, I usually threw them away. If it was a doctor giving me his opinion based on statistics, I would examine the source of the statistics. If it was something that didn't pertain to me, I still might store it in my brain as an interesting fact, but I did not accept it and I did not OWN it. Even if it might pertain to me, I was the one who decided whether or not I would accept it as such. But that still did not mean it was true for me; God and/or I would decide that. What are the words and statements of "fact" that people have spoken to you that you want to remove from your brain store and consciousness?

MIND.BODY

_____

_____

_____

_____

_____

_____

_____

MIND.BODY

_____

_____

_____

_____

_____

_____

_____

_____

_____

_____

_____

_____

_____

_____

_____

_____

What is some of the information that you want to store for yourself and others?

_____

_____

_____

_____

_____

_____

_____

_____

_____

_____

_____

_____

_____

_____

What is some of the "stinking thinking" that you want to rid yourself of?

MIND.BODY

_____

_____

_____

_____

_____

_____

_____

_____

_____

_____

_____

The power of your mind should be consistently exercised over the cancer.

CHAPTER XII

Immunity

*I*magine the old-fashioned teeter-totter. The way things should be is that the immune system is strong enough to weigh down the teeter-totter and hold cancer up in the air. When cancer shows up, it is a clear indication that your immune system is either too busy doing other things or too weakened to hold off the cancer. Strengthening the immune system is of vital importance. The gut—the large and small intestine—is the seat of the immune system. The immune system has huge power in relation to cancer.[26] Cancer's causes are debated, but everyone will agree that a strong immune system is our very best defense against cancer.

One of the best books I've read on ME is by Jesse Stoff, M.D., entitled *Chronic Fatigue Syndrome: The Hidden Epidemic*. I had no idea the immune system had so much involvement with just about every disease. When I read the book after my ME diagnosis, I realized I had great information but that I could do nothing with it because so few doctors in the early 1990s had this level of understanding. Today, thank goodness, the light bulb has gone off for a lot of people. Dr. Stoff says we have to think big picture when understanding the immune system:

> All diseases, either acute and severe or chronic, have, to some degree, an element of immune dysfunction that is central to the

26 http://www.cancerresearch.org/cancer-immunotherapy/resources/cancer-and-the-immune-system

disease process. The immune system is one of our primary and most critical systems, and helps to regulate our internal disease-fighting environment. It exerts its control by virtue of a multitude of circulating components, some of which include cytokines that are capable of acting at sites far removed from their points of origin. Its complexity rivals that of the nervous system, and in fact the similarities between the two are quite real. Cells of the immune system and the nervous system have many hormone receptor sites in common. It is no accident of nature that the thymus gland, the bone marrow, and the lymph nodes—all major centers of immune activity—are bundled in ropes of nerves. The brain is known to transmit both electrical and chemical signals along nerves to stimulate, amplify and modify the immune responses. As the signals stream out from the brain, they often pass warnings from the immune centers flying in the opposite direction. The immune system is not merely a tool that is manipulated by the brain, but rather it is a sensory organ as well. It transmits chemical messages about bacteria, fungi, viruses, bits of dead tissue, and cancer cells. The wonder of it all is that such organization is possible, with the use of only a few distinct cell types whose members are widely scattered throughout the body.

There are some easy and accessible immunotherapies available to everyone. Acupuncture, laughter, loving touch, massage, classical music, and unconditional love (pets) all boost the immune system. Endorphins are anti-cancer and immune-boosting. Let's look at a few of these.

Acupuncture

Most acupuncture treatments involve using ultra-thin needles to penetrate the skin to relieve pain and stimulate proper energy flow in the body. Acupuncture is often used as an adjunct to conventional care and can lead to improvements in quality of life and alleviation of cancer treatment-related side effects. Research shows that acupuncture treatments can increase the body's T-cell count (a component of the immune system), as well as the number of immune cells that ingest and destroy bacteria, protozoa, and cell debris. In one study, for example, patients who received 30 minutes of acupuncture daily for 10 days had higher natural killer (NK) cell activity in their blood compared to the control group.[27] A 2015 animal study found that acupuncture turns off (downregulates) pro-inflammatory cells known as M1 macrophages.[28]

Acupuncture is a form of Traditional Chinese Medicine (TCM), which originated over 2,500 years ago in China. The idea is that an invisible life force called qi (pronounced chee) travels up and down the body in 14 meridians. Illness and pain are due to blockages and imbalances in those meridians. The acupuncture points are thought to have electrical properties, which affect chemical neurotransmitters in the body. Doppler ultrasound shows that acupuncture increases blood flow in treated areas. Thermal imaging shows that it can make inflammation subside. This kind of documentation led to its acceptance by Western medicine; insurance often covers it now.

Laughter[29]

According to some schools of thought, laughter operates on at least three different levels: biophysical, the biochemical, and the bioenergetic levels.

- On the biophysical level, laughter moves lymph fluid around your body simply by the convulsions you experience during the process of laughing. This boosts immune system function and helps clear out old, dead waste products from organs and tissues.

- Laughter increases oxygenation and boosts circulation, so at the same time that you're distributing oxygen around your body, you're

27 Wu B, Zhou RX, Zhou MS. Effect of acupuncture on interleukin-2 level and NK cell immunoactivity of peripheral blood of malignant tumor patients. *Chinese Journal of integrated traditional and Western medicine*, 1994 Sep;14(9):537-9

28 http://www.ncbi.nlm.nih.gov/pubmed/24961568

29 http://www.ncbi.nlm.nih.gov/pmc/articles/PMC2686627

IMMUNITY

boosting the circulation of your blood. You are exercising abdominal muscles. You are exercising the muscles of your face. And, you are enhancing the flexibility of various joints throughout your body. So it's a bit of physical exercise and healthful body movement as well.

- When you laugh, you generate a wealth of healing biochemicals such as serotonin and immune-boosting chemicals such as interleukins. They will boost immune system function. They will improve your outlook on life. They will tend to diminish any symptoms of depression. And because they help reduce stress, they will also reduce all of the various diseases and disorders that are caused by chronic stress.

Now, I realize you don't feel much like laughing when you are dealing with cancer. Even after reading about the healing power of laughter, it was very hard for me to find anything funny. It took me a while trying different comedies on TV until I came across *I Love Lucy* reruns; they made me laugh every time. When I had gone through the reruns, I found *Ellen* on TV. She is hilarious to me, and I laughed every day I watched.

Shortly after I was diagnosed, I went to a place called the Optimum Health Institute for a few weeks (more on that in the Nourishment chapter). One of the first things they had us do every day in our morning exercise class was to belly laugh. We had to stand there and laugh at absolutely nothing for a few minutes. Do you know what? Laughing at absolutely nothing is so contagiously funny that you almost cannot stop laughing!

Endorphins

Endorphins enhance our immune system: When endorphins are secreted, they activate natural killer cells (NK cells) and thereby boost our immune system. Under stress, the competency of our immune system is reduced remarkably. NK cells are likely to lose their effect under stress. NK cells, which take responsibility for the immune system by killing defective cells, also have the ability to kill cancer cells.

There are many things that boost endorphins, such as:

- Exercise
- Acupuncture
- Laughter
- Loving touch
- Belly Breathing (diaphragmatic breathing)
- Sex
- Oral ginseng
- Beetroot
- Sniffing vanilla or lavender
- Chocolate/Cacao
- Avocados
- Music
- Spicy foods
- Meditation
- Brazil nuts (3 per day)
- Daily sunshine (or equivalent vitamin D levels from supplements, fish, fish liver oils, egg yolks)
- Vitamin B boosters
  - B6 for the central nervous system, for the production of dopamine, serotonin, and norepinephrine
  - B9 for synthesizing and regulating neurotransmitters
  - B12 for brain boosting
- Eggs
  - Contain tyrosine as well as tryptophan, plenty of B vitamins and vitamin D that all contribute to producing positive thinking
- Affirmations
- And, last but not least, knitting has been shown to boost endorphins. Yes, knitting.

Loving Touch and Massage

CNN reports:

> Recently, researchers measured immune function in healthy adults who got either a 45 minute Swedish massage or 45 minutes of lighter touch. The massaged group had substantially more white blood cells—including natural killer cells, which help the body fight viruses and other pathogens—and fewer types of inflammatory cytokines associated with autoimmune diseases.[30]

Loving touch can be as simple as a hug, or touching or rubbing someone's back. More formal therapies besides massage include Laying On of Hands or Reiki.

Music

Researchers from Drexel University reviewed 30 trials with a total of 1,891 participants. They included music therapy sessions with a trained music therapist and recorded music played by medical staff. Selections included relaxing music in categories that included classical, jazz, folk, rock, country and western, easy listening, new age, big band, Spanish, and religious. The researchers were able to scientifically measure a significant improvement in anxiety and mood. They were also able to measure small improvements in heart rate, respiratory rate, blood pressure and pain.[31]

Dr. Constantine "Gus" Kotsanis (www.KotsanisInstitite.com) says there are two types of music: anaplastic and dysplastic. "Anaplastic is healing music and psycho-immunity supportive. In this music, the high sound is on the first note; an example would be Beethoven's Ninth Symphony.

---

30 http://www.cnn.com/2011/HEALTH/01/05/touching.makes.you.healthier. health/index.html

31 Bradt, J et al. Music Interventions for Improving Psychological and Physical Outcomes in Cancer Patients. *Cochrane Database of Systematic Reviews* 2011 Aug 10;(8):CD006911. doi: 10.1002/14651858.CD006911.pub2.

The other type is dysplastic which is destructive to the immune system and to the psycho-immunity. Here the high sound is on the third note and repeats itself every third note. An example of this is modern rock music. Of great interest is Byzantine music where the humming of the chanters activates the brain that talks to the Divine.

Also, if you want to program a nation of people, you must do them ideally in German; in the German language the repeated sound is every 17 syllables. If, on the other hand, you do not want to program a nation of people, you talk to them ideally in Greek. What is fascinating about the Greek language is the fact the entire brain is activated by speech. This is in contrast to the German language where not all of the brain is activated by speech."

Supplements

Dr. Bradford Weeks, retired, reported a list of supplements for the immune system at the 2012 BAFC Integrative Oncology Conference:

1. Theanine (increases interferon gamma)
2. Arginine (increases NKC and T-cell function)
3. American ginseng (increases T-cell function)
4. Melatonin (increases IL-2, epidermal growth factor)
5. Thymrevit (increases T-cell function)
6. Vitamin A, C and others
7. Aromatase inhibitors: BioDim, Myomin

I also like to support the immune system by supporting the liver because it has a big job to do, including the majority of our detoxification processes. So get a good liver support supplement. I like Livaplex by Standard Process, but you can only get this from People's Pharmacy or a licensed medical professional, typically a chiropractor. Milk thistle is also good to cleanse and support the liver, but may not be strong enough. You can also try some liver cleanses, but be sure to do extensive research and consult some experienced medical professionals before starting.

Unconditional Love (Pets)

Pets can add a wonderful, positive dimension to our lives. They can boost immunity, ward off depression, and lower blood pressure and triglyceride levels. Animals simply make us feel good. They offer us unconditional love in a world that often seems cold, competitive, and lonely. No one loves us more unconditionally than our pet. It only takes a few minutes with a fuzzy friend to feel less anxious, less stressed. Our body actually goes through physical changes in that time that make a difference in our mood. The level of cortisol, a hormone associated with stress, is lowered. And the production of serotonin, a chemical associated with well-being, is increased.

In my case, it's even more than that. My beloved dog Chia alerts me to when my blood sugar levels get dangerously high. Very low blood sugar causes chemical changes in the human body that give off a scent. When Chia picks up on that, she will get my attention by any means possible—jump up and slap my leg, or lick my face if I am sleeping to wake me up.

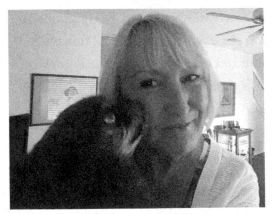

This is a fun platform key to play with. If we have pets, we already know how good they make us feel, with their unconditional acceptance. Notice how good it makes you feel to hug and be hugged or to get a massage.

Because of the ME, I cannot walk or stand for long periods of time so it takes a wheelchair to navigate airports. Since I do not get out of the wheelchair, I do pat-downs at security. Honestly, I now know how my dog feels when I pet her! When I read about knitting creating endorphins, I joined a knitting group, a Prayer Shawl Ministry. What a great time that turned out to be, and I made so many friends! It was a true therapy session, and I was thrilled to be part of it.

Use this space to record your thoughts and intentions on how you are going to make your immune system stronger and more balanced.

_____

_____

_____

_____

_____

_____

IMMUNITY

_____

_____

_____

_____

_____

_____

_____

_____

_____

_____

_____

_____

_____

_____

CHAPTER XIII

Nourishment

*W*e're talking foods, supplementation, herbs, enzymes: everything that can nourish, strengthen, and repair the body at the cellular level.

Foods

Diet is a key part of this modality and serves as a platform for the other aspects. I now know that "you are what you eat" to a very large extent. The basic things to look for in a good diet are: organic; no sugar; fresh; locally-grown if possible; good fats; lots of vegetables high in minerals and fiber; grass-fed meat and pastured eggs; and no MSG or any of those chemical preservatives, additives, and stabilizers whose names we cannot pronounce.

Is there anything more controversial than diet these days? There are many anti-cancer diets out there; choose one that resonates with you. A good basic diet is presented in the book *Beating Cancer with Nutrition* by Dr. Patrick Quillin. He categorizes foods from best anti-cancer to worst. You choose your foods from those categories. He has a handy "cheat sheet" table of foods from best to worst that you can post on your refrigerator or keep in your wallet. Here are a few of other classic cancer diets out there:

Dr. Johanna Budwig's diet is comprised of flax oil, flax seed, and cottage cheese; it is easy, inexpensive, and tasty. You can read about it here and download the free recipe http://www.budwigcenter.com/the-budwig-diet/#.VttKNOZSJIw. This diet has been touted to help reverse many disease states. I heard about it a lot back in 2001, but I don't hear much about it anymore. My understanding is that the flax is meant to provide oxygen to the cells. Cancer cannot survive in an oxygen-rich environment. But along came Wendy Sellens, a Chinese Medicine doctor, who makes a compelling argument against flax: Flooding our bodies with plant-based estrogens is not a good thing, especially since 80 percent of breast cancers are fueled with estrogen. Most women today are estrogen-dominant, and flax "is actually the strongest plant estrogen. Soy has 8,000 units of phytoestrogens per 1/4 cup, while flax is 20 times stronger with 163,000 units of phytoestrogens."[32]

How's that for controversy? I no longer eat flax. Dr. John Young of St. Petersburg, Florida, has enhanced the Budwig shake with protein powder, fish oil, and alkaline boosting drops. http://www.youngfoundationalhealth.com/young-power-shake

The Gerson Therapy has been effective for many. A friend of mine had breast cancer in 1997. She had a lumpectomy and went on the Gerson diet. She always felt that the diet, combined with supplements, helped her get through radiation therapy with no side effects. Here is the Gerson Institute website http://gerson.org/gerpress/the-gerson-therapy/ for more information.

Macrobiotic diets are also popular with patients who are seeking to heal or to live a healthier lifestyle. There is a great deal out there on the internet about macrobiotics; here is a good overall review of the origins and components: https://en.wikipedia.org/wiki/Macrobiotic_diet.

The blood type diet. Eat according to your nutritional type. The potent anti-cancer effects of this principle are very much underappreciated. Dr. Peter J. D'Adamo's book *Eat Right 4 Your Type* has a simple, effective formula: 4 blood types; 4 individual diet plans.

---

32 Sellens W. A Flax Fairytale. Accessed at http://abreastboutique.com/blogs/breast-darn-thermography-blog-ever-this-aint-your-mothers-breast-screening/17883365-the-flax-fairytale-f-flax-and-the-horse-it-rode-in-on

- Blood Type O thrives on a lean, high protein diet.
- Blood Type A thrives on a primarily vegetarian diet.
- Blood Type B thrives on a mixed diet of meat, fish and dairy.
- Blood Type AB thrives on a modified vegetarian diet.

I'm an A+ but until I got cancer I did not eat many vegetables. I appreciate them more now because organic vegetables taste delicious, but I still don't stay on any diet very long as I am devoted to fooling the cancer and not letting it get immune to anything.

The Paleo diet has become very popular in the last several years. Basically, the idea is that we should eat like our ancestors, meaning nutrient dense food that comes as God made it, not as man has manufactured it. The theory is that this diet will keep your and your genome healthy because you will avoid added sugars, carcinogenic pesticides, man-made industrial fats, refined and hybridized grains, and processed foods. Ancestral diets are estimated to have been 20- to 40 percent carbohydrates, 15- to 30 percent protein, and up to 65 percent fat.

You can find some good information on the diet, research/science, and recipes here http://robbwolf.com/what-is-the-paleo-diet and here http://www.marksdailyapple.com.

This is the diet that I primarily adhere to. A common misconception of the "paleo diet" is that it is all meat. It's not. If you eat, say, three handfuls of vegetables for every handful protein, it's a good all-around anti-cancer diet, and easy to stick to. It has also been shown to lower blood sugar, which means that it is very good for diabetes as well as cancer.

The term "Paleo" has evolved over time to where it now encompasses a holistic approach that somewhat mirrors the hunter-gatherer lifestyle. So you will often see Paleo advocates emphasizing getting enough sleep at night, moving throughout the day, and reducing stress levels.

The Ketogenic diet was created by a doctor at the Mayo Clinic in 1924 for treating epilepsy. Despite its success, it fell out of fashion in the 1940s due to the advent of seizure medication. (Profit triumphs over natural remedies yet again.)

Ketogenic researcher Dr. Dominic D'Agostino says, "Sugar addiction is the Achilles heel of cancer cells" and the ketogenic diet is a low, low sugar diet. It relies on using ketones for energy instead of glucose. Ketones are formed with the body breaks down fat for fuel. Cancer cells need a constant supply of glucose to stay alive but normal cells can use ketones as an alternative fuel whereas cancer cells cannot. Ketogenic diets lower that all important blood glucose level which effectively starves cancer cells while nourishing normal cells.

The Standard American Diet is high sugar—either the kind easily recognized in sodas and cupcakes, or in the so-called *other* sugar, starchy carbs like bread and pasta and cereal that quickly convert into sugar in the body. Over time, our bodies adapt and we become sugar burners. Yet our body is designed to burn fat as its primary fuel. A ketogenic diet is a fat-burning way of eating.

A great book on the diet is *Fight Cancer with a Ketogenic Diet*, an eBook by Ellen Davis, M.S. This is an essential, well referenced book, and it is based on cutting edge research on ketogenic dietary therapies from Dr. Dominic D'Agostino and Dr. Thomas Seyfried at Boston College. It offers 120 pages of the latest information on:

- how and why a low carb, ketogenic diet works to stop cancer cells, how to implement the diet, and how to monitor your progress
- blood glucose and ketone level targets recommended to destroy cancer
- what foods to choose and how much to eat
- why certain foods must be restricted
- use of calorie restriction and fasting
- whether alcohol is allowed
- the debate between acidity vs alkalinity
- appropriate supplementation

Even though my "go-to" diet for the last few years has been the Paleo diet, I have been interested in the keto diet for the anti-cancer aspects as well as the benefits to diabetics. I am currently working with one of Best Answer for Cancer's (BAFC) key physician members, Dr. David Minkoff, in order to investigate the keto diet and assist me in getting on it. If you investigate this diet, be sure to do it under the guidance of a physician who has a good track record with it and a full program to manage it.

And by the way, what is the difference between Paleo and Ketogenic? Both are low-carb, moderate protein, high fat diets. A classic ketogenic diet is 75- to 80 percent fats, mostly medium chain triglycerides, meaning coconut oil and palm kernel oil. It is low protein and low carb, about 10 percent of each. The keto diet's very low carb requirement, just 50 to 80 grams of carbohydrate per day, is so low that some critics say you can't get in enough vegetables (vegetables are a carbohydrate). Paleo is more forgiving. The bottom line is that we are all different; nutritionists call this "bioindividuality." If some of us go too low carb, we can trigger hypothyroidism or have fertility issues.

A raw, organic, vegan diet. Consider a short-term nutritional detox using a raw organic vegetarian diet, wheatgrass juice, and wheatgrass enemas (the Optimum Health Institute Program), which feeds the body at the cellular level and causes the cells to flush toxins. The Hippocrates Health Institute had the first program of this nature, and it remains the premiere holistic lifestyle program. In the last few years, they have included a PsychoNeuroImmunological Program by Dr. Janet Hranicky called the Comprehensive Cancer Wellness Program (CCWP): a mind/body wellness program for cancer and chronic disease. To my way of thinking, the mind/body and spiritual aspects are the missing links to healing all diseases.

I went to the Optimum Health Institute a few weeks after I was diagnosed. They offered a total organic raw vegan diet, heavy juicing, wheatgrass, a whole body cleanse, enemas, colonics, exercise, yoga, food classes and other natural remedies.

I stayed at this clinic for seven weeks, and felt much better. They teach that the order of what you eat is very important. Juices digest most quickly, then fruits, then vegetables. Raw digests first, then cooked.

After the fruits and vegetables, the order of digestion is:

1. Starchy vegetables
2. Grains
3. Starches
4. Fish
5. Chicken
6. Turkey
7. Pork
8. Lamb
9. Venison
10. Bison
11. Beef

If you eat meat, make it organic meat, but eat it last, because it progresses through the digestive system slower than anything else. So if you eat the meat first, then the potato, then the vegetables, the potato and vegetables have to wait for the meat to digest before it goes through your intestinal tract. This means you have food just sitting around and rotting in your digestive tract. Which means more toxins to overload the vital body organs.

Some medical experts argue with this but all I can say is it is my experience that when I eat in this order, I digest very well and my stomach stays flatter. When I eat out of order is when I have bloating and indigestion.

I remained on a raw organic vegan diet for 7½ months. But I did not feel well after that long on the diet. Several different doctors confirmed that I needed animal fats/protein in my diet. But it was not just the doctors' opinions: I *felt* like I needed meat. So I gradually added cooked foods and a little organic meat back into my diet. I felt very good and the scans were showing that the tumors were generally staying the same, but I also had some shrinkage. My current modified Paleo diet of mostly vegetables with a small amount of meat allows me that along with the comfort of certain organic meats still being anti-cancer. (Organic meats do not have hormones, steroids, or antibiotics.)

NOURISHMENT

We hear a great deal about raw organic vegan diets, or just vege-tarian, and how good they are for you. However, most people do not thrive on this diet for long periods of time. Nutritional researchers Loren Cordain and Dr. Weston Price said they never found evidence that any of our historical ancestors, regardless of where they lived in the world, survived on just a vegetarian diet.

As it is right now, I go on and off the diet a few times each year, and for the rest of the time my diet consists of 80 percent raw vegeta-bles and 20 percent cooked vegetables/animal products. For fats I use avocado and coconut oil to sauté, and olive oil for dressing. I also do my best to get organic, grass-fed beef and chicken. I get my eggs from a farmer's market where I know I am getting them from chickens that really had access to free range. I'm not comfortable doing fish anymore because of the contamination. My omega-3s come from chia seeds, eggs, and my grass-fed meats. And I eat nuts.

My personal belief is that if your physical condition will tolerate it, the first diet after diagnosis should be a raw, organic, vegan diet with cleanses/enemas. Raw organic vegetables digest at the cellular level, which causes the cells to push out toxins.

The reason I believe this to be true is due to two experiences I had while at the Optimum Health Institute. The first example was an artist from Florida who came every year to detox: she walked around smelling of turpentine. The second experience had to do with me per-sonally. I'm a militant ex-smoker, and in my third week there, I kept smelling cigarettes. So I went on a mission to find the person who was sneaking cigarettes into this organic, healing environment. One day, I turned back to say something to someone behind me, and I smelled the cigarettes on my arm: I was detoxing nicotine after 16 years! My conclusion was that the diet is a very good way to detox while re-nour-ishing the body at the cellular level.

Dr. Thomas Lodi (http://www.anoasisofhealing.com) is a passion-ate believer in the power of a raw, vegan diet and its influence on our genetics. He says:

It is estimated that we lose and produce 2 to 3 million new cells per second which accounts for the fact that we change the lining to our intestines every 3 days. We have new rod and cones in our retinas every 48 hours, all new skin every 6 weeks and a new liver approximately every 6 months. The raw materials necessary for cellular repair and regeneration as well as the energy to carry out the millions of chemical reactions required every second, are provided by nature in the form of food and water. Each species comes equipped with a specialized anatomy and instinct to eat what is appropriate in order to thrive. We are hominid primates, designed to eat plants (leaves, stems, roots, fruit and seeds). It is only when we eat and live our lives in accordance with our biological requirements, that we can achieve optimal functioning, hence optimal healing.

Check out:

- Hippocrates Health Institute in West Palm Beach, Florida, the original cleanse program that has become a very comprehensive holistic lifestyle program http://hippocratesinst.org

- The Optimum Healthy Institute in Austin, Texas, or San Diego, California http://www.optimumhealth.org

Microbiome (gut flora)

Our bodies are home to some 100 trillion bacteria that have evolved with us. In fact, they outnumber our human cells by 10 to 1. Turns out these bacteria are probably more important in determining our health than the genes we were born with and thus scientists have come to think of them as "the second genome."

The majority of these microbes live in our gut. People who are obese, for example, apparently have a different microbial makeup than people who are not. The sharp rise in autoimmune diseases appears linked to disruptions in our gut microbes from the relatively sterile standard American diet. Research demonstrates that the diversity of bacteria the Western gut is significantly lower than in less-industrialized populations.

NOURISHMENT

There is talk in some circles of "restoration ecology" and fecal implants. We used to eat fermented foods which fed our gut flora, but today, about the only fermented food people eat is the occasional pickle. Sauerkraut is a good place to start. You can buy pre-made kimchee. Raw milk fans make kefir and yogurt (pasteurized, commercial yogurt often is not a good source of probiotics—and most yogurts you can buy are full of sugar). There are lots of good books out there on how to ferment vegetables.

Probiotic supplements get mixed reviews as to whether they provide sufficient diversity and whether they survive the trip through the acid stomach. A prebiotic feeds the process by which bacteria are made rather than just supplementing with a few stains; a prebiotic with which people have reported good results is acacia senegal soluble fiber. Beneficial microorganisms living in our colons have profound effects on our health, including brain development, behavior, memory, and learning.

Supplementation

The average American is said to be painfully low on some important basics: vitamin D, the B vitamins, magnesium, selenium, choline…

Supplements can feed the body, especially if they work at the cellular level like the wild blue green algae that I used from Cell Tech. There are many sources to choose from. Look for one sourced in Klamath Lake, Oregon that includes enzymes.

Intravenous (IV) delivery is a "therapeutic" way to deliver supplements, meaning you can receive bigger doses directly into the blood stream than you can get taking a pill by mouth.

Cancer patients tend to be especially depleted of nutrients so IVs are a good way to go. They can nourish and repair the body and the vital body organs as well as treat cancer and chronic disease. IV vitamin C, for example, is a favorite in cancer clinics because it can kill cancer cells just like chemo, but unlike chemo, people do not build up a resistance to it and there are no toxic side effects other than that over time, it can be hard on the veins. Plus, vitamin C is great at killing viruses and viruses are often involved in the cancer scenario. Vitamin C is a natural detoxifying agent.

A "Myers cocktail" is another favorite IV. Think of it as a super multi-vitamin because it usually includes magnesium, calcium, various B vitamins, vitamin C, and the antioxidant glutathione.

LET, or "liposomal encapsulation technology," started with vitamin C and now more nutrients are available in liposomal form. Curcumin is a favorite. They look like capsules but the nutrient is actually wrapped in a fat membrane which increases its absorption through the gut. Recent research suggests liposomal vitamin C is as effective as the IV. You could say you get more bang for the buck with this delivery system, and no needle required.

A worthwhile test for your roadmap is a blood test from RGCC-USA. The patient has a qualified physician draw their blood, and the blood sample is shipped overnight to Greece. The RGCC lab in Greece tests that sample for sensitivities to different chemotherapies, IV therapies, supplements, and foods. The patient gets back a report showing what will be effective—and what won't—for their individual cancer. This blueprint can help patients plot their Healing Platform more effectively.

Herbs and Spices

Modern processed food relies heavily on salt to make it tasty, which is a shame because herbs are the natural way to add flavor. Plus, they have health benefits:

- Garlic, for example, has a long history of being used medicinally. It has antimicrobial, antiviral, and anti-parasitic activity.

- Turmeric now has more than 500 peer-reviewed studies on it and it looks like a superstar. This is the spice that gives Indian food its yellow-orange color. No matter what chronic disease researchers test it for, turmeric helps. It is a powerful anti-inflammatory, breaks down toxins in the liver, and stimulates the immune system.

- Cumin is extremely good for digestion, accelerates the secretion of detoxifying and anticarcinogenic enzymes, and adding some cumin seed to rice just makes it taste wonderful.

- Fennel contains substances that loosen lung mucus and help clear the chest; research shows that fennel also lowers blood pressure.

- Parsley, fenugreek, cayenne, and marjoram are some herbs loaded with vitamins, antioxidants, and are also cancer-fighting.

Enzymes

Cancer patients tend to have digestive challenges and malabsorption of nutrients. Digestive enzymes help you break down food more completely and assist your body in utilizing necessary vitamins and nutrients.

Systemic enzymes, on the other hand, are taken on an empty stomach. Some 99 percent of the enzymes in our body are systemic. They are the catalysts that put vitamins and minerals to work to speed up chemical reactions. In cancer, the big workhorses are the proteolytic systemic enzymes, meaning they go after protein. Proteolytic enzymes break down excess fibrin that feeds chronic diseases, including cancer. Proteolytic enzymes such as papain, bromelain, serratiopeptidase, and nattokinase are formulated into supplements for healing purposes.

Dr. Nicholas Gonzalez of New York documented the use of enzyme therapy as a cancer therapy. (See the chapter on Targeted Cancer Therapies for more information.) Consider working with a doctor to choose the correct enzyme therapy for you.

Note in closing

It is important to switch things around in this modality. Avoid patterns of food, supplements, herbs, IV therapies, etc. Remember that cancer is smart, and like a weed, it wants to survive; it wants to build immunities against things it senses threaten its survival.

For my supplement chart in my Healing Platform, I had start and stop dates for every supplement, and there were no patterns. For instance, I would take something for four weeks and then switch to something else for six weeks, and then to something else for three weeks. With all diets, I made sure I did not eat the same things all the time. I would choose different vegetables every time I went grocery shopping.

KEEP CANCER ON ITS TOES!
NEVER LET IT SEE YOU COMING!

NOURISHMENT

Your diet now needs to become a way of life. Survivor research shows that most survivors do not go through cancer and then go back to their previous lifestyle. You have to remember that your previous lifestyle probably contributed to feeding the cancer. This is especially true of diet. The standard American diet contains many addictive foods, especially processed foods formulated with sugar, oil-based industrial fats, and too generous amounts of refined salt. Food manufacturers go to great lengths to encourage us to eat more, to buy more of these oh-so-tasty foods that are often high in calories, and very low in nutrition. As you let go of these processed foods, your brain may scream for them, especially for sugar. But ignore it. After 2-3 weeks, the screaming will be over. It's generally easier if you go cold turkey instead of trying to wean yourself off them.

Certain tenets will always hold true as an anti-cancer approach, such as avoiding all sugar. But in other areas, it is good to switch around your food choices, both to avoid boredom and to expose yourself to new vegetables, new proteins, new herbs, and the healing compounds they contain. But don't forget that cancer builds immunities against things. So keep switching things around.

The strictness of the diet can flex, too, as long as it does not ever get too lax. As Dr. Quillin says, if you drop down every once in a blue moon to the "Worst" category for anti-cancer foods, don't beat yourself up. Just get back up into the "Best" category as soon as possible.

Decide on your beginning diet. Note the books you want to buy. Then buy them, read them, and make notes about how you want to proceed. Don't forget about buying your items through AMAZON SMILE. Nonprofits receive a small percentage of any/all sales using this link: www.amazon.com/ch/20-5469118. Keep us handy for all your shopping!

After you have done your research on the options in this modality, carefully decide your schedule of start and stop dates for each method you employ. You will want to stagger the intervals. For instance, you might want to do one diet or supplement for 3 weeks and then get off for 4 weeks, doing a different diet or supplement for those 4 weeks but then getting off that one for 6 weeks. Be careful not to have any patterns that cancer can anticipate. Always keep cancer unaware. "Never let it see you coming!" Then GO!

NOURISHMENT

_____

_____

_____

_____

_____

_____

_____

_____

NOURISHMENT

NOURISHMENT

CHAPTER XIV

Detox

A diagnosis of cancer typically signifies a toxic overload. Toxins can be:

- Environmental—air pollution, water contaminants and additives like fluoride, building materials and furniture that off gas chemicals, electro-magnetic frequencies that disturb our natural cell-to-cell communication, perfumes made with petrochemicals, personal care products with suspected or known carcinogens, cleaning products, air fresheners.

- Physical—food is the big one here, and lack of exercise factors in too because movement keeps our lymph system moving and prompts us to make good neurotransmitters.

- As well as spiritual, emotional, psychological, and intellectual.

According to chemical analysis of 10 umbilical cord blood samples from newborns, 287 toxins were identified in umbilical cords, 180 of which cause cancer.[33] So we are immersed, in the womb even, in a chemically-saturated environment. Then we add to our toxic exposures and overload as we grow older.

The Center for Disease Control's 2009 report of blood, serum, and urine samples from 2500 random participants showed that all

---

33 http://www.ewg.org/research/body-burden-pollution-newborns

Americans are recipients of widespread exposure to environmental chemicals. This ranges from BPA and lead, to acrylamides in fried food and gasoline additives.[34]

Environmental

According to the President's Cancer Panel report released in 2010:

> With the growing body of evidence linking environmental exposures to cancer, the public is becoming increasingly aware of the unacceptable burden of cancer resulting from environmental and occupational exposures that could have been prevented through appropriate national action ... The Panel was particularly concerned to find that the true burden of environmentally induced cancer has been grossly underestimated.[35]

So environmental carcinogens are all around us, and in many ways, we are on our own when it comes to limiting our exposure to them. That report is worth reading because, as government reports go, it is surprisingly candid and easy to read.

Let's look at some of the big challenges:

A. *Air.* Air pollution is linked to heart disease, lung cancer and acute and chronic respiratory conditions, such as asthma. Get air purifiers like Fresh Air Classic from Vollara that treat VOCs and the following toxins:

1. Building products (paint, glues, varnish, flooring, countertops, carpeting, walls)
2. Manufactured products (cars/vehicles, toys, cooking utensils and other household items)
3. Furniture, clothing/linens

DETOX

---

34 Fourth National Report on Human Exposure to Environmental Chemicals, CDC, 2009. Accessed at http://www.cdc.gov/exposurereport

35 2008–2009 Annual President's Cancer Panel Report, "Reducing Environmental Cancer Risk." Accessed at http://deainfo.nci.nih.gov/advisory/pcp/annualReports/pcp08-09rpt/PCP_Report_08-09_508.pdf

4. Cleaning products

5. Perfumes, air fresheners, wax candles

6. Dust and dust mites

7. Animal dander

8. Molds, mildew

9. Viruses, bacteria

My go-to source for Vollara is Carl Thompson at Enviromed Sciences. He can be contacted at Carl@Enviromedsciences.com.

B. *Water.* Get water purifiers and filters for all household water. Tests have shown that water sold in plastic bottles is not always as filtered as we would like, and most likely it has an endocrine-disrupting chemical in it called Bisphenol A (BPA). Be on the lookout also for Bisphenol S (BPS) or any members of this chemical family; when mommy-bloggers revolted against BPA's gender-bending qualities, many manufacturers of plastic bottles quietly switched to related chemicals. You may see "BPA-Free" on the label, but that doesn't mean it wasn't made with BPS. Your safest alternative is glass or stainless steel. You can read more about BPA here: http://www.breastcancerfund.org/clear-science/radiation-chemicals-and-breast-cancer/bisphenol-a.html I suggest that you fill your own bottle with purified water and take with you.

Carbon-based systems will remove most of the chlorine, and that's a big help. Chlorine creates THMs and haloforms, potent chemical pollutants that create excess free radicals which lead to cell damage. A whole house water filter is best because our skin is the largest organ, and showering in chorine water is no different than drinking it.

At the kitchen sink where you draw water for cooking and drinking, consider a reverse osmosis (RO) system. An RO system can also remove fluoride; carbon-based systems cannot because fluoride is a very small molecule. Although the "fluoride is good for teeth" myth has been unraveling over the years, and studies show that 41 percent of teens in the U.S. exhibit dental fluorosis (too much fluoride), most municipal water systems still add it.

Phillippe Grandjean, an expert in environmental toxins, puts the risk of fluoride right up there with other brain toxins like lead and mercury. A study by the Environmental Protection Agency found that long-term high intake of fluoride can increase the risk of brittle bones and fractures. Additionally, fluoride poisons hundreds of enzymes in the body, plays havoc with the thyroid gland, and has been linked to cancer. It's worth getting fluoride out of your water.

RO water does not have minerals in it, but if you have a nutrient dense diet, that won't be an issue. Also, RO systems generate waste water. Depending upon the system, about 5 gallons discharge to the sewer system for every 1 gallon of drinking water created. Pure water is not produced without a cost, no matter what the technology.

My Vollara water purifier gives me alkaline, purified, and acidic water. I drink the alkaline during the day away from meals. If I drink during meals, I use the purified water. I use the acidic water for washing my face, my pots and pans, and watering my plants.

NOTE: Do not ever buy alkaline water in a bottle from the store, because water cannot hold an alkaline charge for long (even in a glass container), therefore it is a waste of money.

C. Electro-magnetic fields (EMFs) and the ionizing radiation from X-rays and medical scans come at us in much greater magnitudes today than in our parents' generation. There is no disagreement that ionizing radiation causes cancer; yet no one keeps track of how much exposure we get through various X-rays. The CT scan, for example, is notorious for its heavy exposure to X-rays. Doctors are quick to sell us the whiz-bang of the pictures a scan will generate, but we need to consider the downside of the ionizing radiation because it is carcinogenic.

DETOX

Cell phones, utility smart meters, and wireless networks are non-ionizing radiation. Most industry-sponsored studies find this EMF exposure safe and most independent studies do not. It's very much a case of consumer beware in the marketplace. A great resource to educate yourself on this is: http://www.bioinitiative.org.

There are many EMF blockers/neutralizers on the market. These range from dots you put on your cell phone and laptop, to EMF blocking paint and bed screening material. Some work better than others.

I have found that we all have different sensitivities to energy. For example, some people report they feel so woozy and nauseous after a utility company installs a smart meter that they can barely function. Other people report a wide range of effects including headaches, tinnitus, insomnia, heart palpitations, memory issues, or fatigue. In my experience, I find it is very much an acquired skill to learn how you react to it and how you feel when it is neutralized. I can actually feel the difference when I have my EMF neutralizer on. I feel calmer, with a sense of "smoothness": there is no jittery feeling. And I am less aggressive in the car.

Many people find it helpful to replace the cordless phones in their homes with corded phones. Turning off printers until you need to use them can reduce EMF fields in your office. Do you really need a wireless mouse or will a corded mouse do just as well? Can you use the speaker on your cell phone instead of holding it next to your head? And can you not park that cell phone in your bra or hip pocket? My point is that despite the convenience of our wireless world, we are surrounded now with these man-made energy emissions that appear to want to break our DNA and alter our cell membrane permeability. We can practice avoidance to minimize our exposure.

DETOX

Physical

A. *Detox*—Our bodies are designed to detox. However, the body struggles to detox the copious amount of stuff thrown at it in the modern environment. Plus, the standard American diet leaves us malnourished in terms of vitamins, minerals, enzymes, and co-factors that our bodies need for the job of detoxification. There are an estimated 80,000 chemicals in our environment, most of which have never been tested for safety. Tests show that the widely used herbicide glyphosate shows up in our blood and urine, for example. And on it goes. We can help the immune system stay focused on its primary mission by supporting it with detox programs. There are a number of options for this including a multi-day juice fast, saunas, and making use of cleanses targeted at various organ systems.

The colon, the last part of our large intestine, is where most cleansing programs start because you want to make sure that you can excrete (poop out) what you target for elimination. Many people like to combine supplements designed for this with a series of colonics, a gentle rinsing of the large intestine with pure water. A professional colon therapist can also make use of organic coffee to stimulate the gall bladder to flush out bile, and thus create fresh bile which we need to digest fats. People who have been on a low-fat diet often have a sluggish gall bladder. The colon is an absorbent organ so sometimes therapists also can make use of wheatgrass, chlorella, and other detoxifying agents by implanting those at the end of the session (you hold it as long as you can).

Heavy metals are increasing in our environment and can build up in the body, poisoning metabolic pathways and allowing pathogens to build biofilms to shield themselves from the immune system. For example, there are issues of arsenic contaminating rice and chicken, mercury in tuna and dental fillings, cadmium in batteries and cigarette smoke, and lead in air and food. Chelation is a proven method for removing heavy metals from the body. It

DETOX

involves intravenous injections of the chelating agent EDTA (ethylene diamine tetra-acetic acid), a synthetic amino acid that binds to heavy metals and excretes them via the urine.

The key to any cleansing-type of detoxification program is to actually get the contaminates out, rather than liberate them and allow them to re-distribute. It's advisable to work with a doctor who has expertise in this area.

B. *Exercise*—You've probably heard the expression that "sitting is the new smoking." Dr. James Levine who coined that phrase says prolonged sitting increases the risk of serious illnesses including cancer, heart disease, and type 2 diabetes. Our bodies were meant to move. I watched my parents lose muscle tone as they aged and reduced their movement. I remember saying to them: "If you don't use it, you will lose it."

Note: Studies show that hard core cardio is not good for us because the body sees that as a stress and releases the stress hormone cortisol, which is part of the reason why so many people do not lose weight primarily with exercise; control of their weight metabolism comes primarily with diet. Our need to move is not so much about an intense hour at the gym as it is a constant amount of movement throughout the day that uses our muscles (leg muscles especially) and keeps our circulation moving and burns up the sugar in our blood stream which in turn calls upon the body to burn more fat.

TAKE ACTION:

- Walk up the stairs instead of taking the elevator.
- Don't park in the spot nearest to the shopping center entrance.
- Take a walk around the block when you get home after work.
- If you spend a lot of time at the desk, get up every hour and move for 5 minutes.

DETOX

Spiritual

Think about finding a higher power or entity that feels larger and more powerful than you. Even if you don't succeed, the experience may offer an expansion of your mindset in that area. Get rid of suspicions, anger, resentment, bitterness, toxic emotions against and about God. I did counseling for this as well as a great deal of journaling. These aspects, along with the Emotional, are two of the biggest hidey-holes for our diseases. We typically "don't want to go there" but the rewards for clearing these areas are immense.

Emotional

Purge toxic memories; get rid of guilt, bitterness, anger, resentment, sadness, negative emotions, and trauma residue that can go as far back as childhood. Tools for this include counseling, self-help books, 12-step programs like Al-Anon, Emotional Recall Healing, Neural Emotional Therapy, Emotional Freedom Technique (EFT), Eye Movement Desensitization Reprocessing (EMDR), and simple old-fashioned crying inspired by sad books and movies.

Most oncologists are not comfortable poking around in people's emotions. It's easier to promote chemo/surgery/radiation and compliment them on their wig. But doctors and staff should be talking emotions, and here's why: The CDC states that 85 percent of disease is caused by emotions. It is likely that this factor may be more important than all the other physical ones listed here, so make sure this is addressed.

Also supportive of this is the 1998 Adverse Childhood Events (ACE) Study,[36] which explained how childhood experiences, both positive and negative, have a tremendous impact on lifelong health and opportunity.

---

36 Felitti V, Anda RF et al. Relationship of Childhood Abuse and Household Dysfunction to Many of the Leading Causes of Death in Adults. *American Journal of Preventative Medicine*, Volume 14, Issue 4 , Pages 245-258, May 1998

My particular favorite tool for this purpose is the Emotional Freedom Technique (see more at http://eft.mercola.com); I have used all of the above methods and continue to go to Al-Anon regularly.

Psychological

The American Cancer Society states:

> Research has shown that psychotherapy may improve a patient's quality of life. It can help reduce anxiety and depression that sometimes occur in people with cancer. It can also help people cope with cancer and the changes in their lives.[37]

Negative thinking simply is not healthy. It increases our stress levels and that can trigger a cascade of chemicals to be released in our bodies that down regulates our immune system and the function of other organs. Cancer patients tend to struggle with issues of self-confidence and self-love. Some helpful tools are:

- Counseling
- Self-help books
- 12-step programs like Al-Anon (a support group for friends and families of problem drinkers and substance abusers)
- Emotional Freedom Technique (EFT—a therapeutic psychological tool that involves tapping acupressure points; learn about it at http://eft.mercola.com)
- Eye Movement Desensitization Reprocessing (EMDR—a psychotherapy treatment originally designed to alleviate distress associated with traumatic memories; learn about it at www.emdr.com). The EMDR method was especially helpful to me in dealing with psychological traumas resulting from an abusive husband.

Note how some of these tools can be used for different approaches and different issues.

DETOX

37 http://www.cancer.org/treatment/treatmentsandsideeffects/
complementaryandalternativemedicine/mindbodyandspirit/psychotherapy

Your Mission

Detox is a very comprehensive modality and one you will spend a great deal of time on. You will not need start or stop times here, either. Detox should be continual for the rest of your life. You want to keep your body, mind, and spirit as clean as possible so as not to feed the cancer with any toxins or negatives and also so as not to tax your immune system.

Journaling is a great method to help identify toxic emotions, thoughts, and physical ailments before they become "dis-ease."

For each aspect of detox, list your approaches/therapies/tools.

Environmental:

_____

_____

_____

_____

_____

_____

_____

_____

_____

_____

_____

_____

_____

DETOX

Physical:

_____

_____

_____

_____

_____

_____

_____

_____

_____

_____

_____

_____

_____

_____

DETOX

Spiritual:

_____

_____

_____

_____

_____

_____

_____

_____

_____

_____

_____

_____

_____

DETOX

Emotional:

_____

_____

_____

_____

_____

_____

_____

_____

_____

_____

_____

_____

_____

_____

DETOX

Psychological:

_____

_____

_____

_____

_____

_____

_____

_____

_____

_____

_____

_____

_____

_____

DETOX

DETOX

_____

_____

_____

_____

_____

_____

_____

_____

_____

_____

_____

_____

_____

_____

_____

_____

_____

CHAPTER XV

Lifestyle

*R*emember: This is the first day of the rest of your life. Literally, the first day of the rest of your life is the day you are born. But it doesn't really become real to us until we hear, "I'm sorry, it's cancer." At that point, our mortality is no longer a concept sometime in the future. It is real, it is now, and it feels like it is *right in your face*.

So, whether you end up living into your 90s or whether you die tomorrow in a car accident, ***this is the first day of the rest of your life.***

Which begs the questions:

- How do I want to live?
- How do I want to die?

One study reported in *Harvard Men's Health* shows lifestyle changes have beneficial impact on cancer patients.[38] Cancer Research UK reports that, "Experts estimate that more than 4 in 10 cancer cases could be prevented by lifestyle changes."[39]

Recreate your lifestyle. Get rid of stress and negatives. Look for ways to make life serene, positive, and fulfilling. Are you sleeping 7-8 hours each night? Stop sleeping during the day and examine all depressive activities. If you are depressed, anxious, and stressed (most cancer

---

38 *Harvard Men's Health Watch*, July 2007

39 http://www.cancerresearchuk.org/cancer-info/healthyliving/introducingcancerprevention/can-cancer-be-prevented

patients are), a good book is *The Mood Cure* by Julia Ross with which you can create a nutritherapy plan to address your issues.

Are you exercising? Qigong, yoga, tai chi, and walking are all good low-impact, low-stress exercise techniques. Walking for 35 minutes each day is a great and easy exercise; a brisk walk is gentle on the body and creates endorphins that are anti-depressant and anti-cancer.

You can also combine aspects of different modalities. For instance, when I walk I also do a visualization technique where I breathe in the power of God and exhale the dis-ease, sending it back to God. Recreate your lifestyle. Examine your lifestyle critically. Do you enjoy life? Are you happy? Are you getting enough rest and relaxation? Are you sleeping well?

You can do a lot, right now, to significantly decrease your cancer risk or to treat active cancer. Even the conservative American Cancer Society states that one-third of cancer deaths are linked to poor diet, physical inactivity, and carrying excess weight. So making the following healthy lifestyle changes can go a very long way toward ending the failure-streak and becoming one less statistic in this war against cancer:

Eliminate negatives (people, situations). When I started examining where, when, and with whom I felt negative, it was very easy to identify what I needed to change. But some of those negative people were relatives! I made the decision to tell each one that I needed their positive support and that if they could not give it to me, I would have to stop seeing them for a while. Most made the adjustment, but there were some friends and family I had to back away from. I had to believe increasing my chances of survival outweighed hurting their feelings.

Reduce and/or control stress. Stress has an impact at the cellular level, and it is believed to be a precursor to disease. Stress reduction and control is still probably my biggest challenge, and I do not think I am alone in this as a cancer patient. But it *can* be done; it is just a constant activity in my life to do things to reduce stress. I took the tools:

- meditation and relaxation techniques
- self-hypnosis
- belly breathing (see below)

And either used them by themselves or combined them with all the previous therapies, imagery, and visualization. I always try to switch it up, to keep the cancer on its toes.

Most recently, I heard about NuCalm, and I bought a system to use for my healing. NuCalm is a way to balance the autonomic nervous system. It calms and focuses your mind while your body recovers. You can read more about it at www.nucalm.com.

Participate in fun activities. If you are like me, you are saying something like, "What in the world could be fun right now?" It may be difficult to find something to make you laugh or enjoy yourself, but you must keep on trying. If you are weak, start slow with TV comedy oldies such as *I Love Lucy, The Carol Burnett Show, The Honeymooners, M.A.S.H., Bewitched,* and many more. You can find most of these on cable TV channels, some on Amazon, and nearly all on the Internet Movie Database (IMDb). When I felt strong enough physically, I took my dog to the dog park and watched her play with others. I would also go to shelters and offer to walk the dogs or play with the cats. In the last few years, I have found group TV parties that are fun such as: sports watching parties, bachelor/bachelorette watching, and Academy Awards parties.

Positive support groups. When I was first diagnosed, I was encouraged to join a support group. So off I went to my oncologist's most highly-recommended group which was my HMO's breast cancer support group. After three meetings of listening to other patients' woes and troubles and recurrences and divorce/death stories, I had definitely had it with that sort of support group. I wanted people around me who would encourage, challenge, and praise me. I ended up joining a Prayer Shawl Ministry: a group of people who got together and made shawls for the sick, infusing them with prayer during their creation. I also joined a new divorcees group where newly single men and women got together to bolster each other in their new and re-emerging social skills.

Count your blessings. Every night, the last thing before I go to bed, I count my blessings. My goal is to count at least 10. It's funny, but I rarely get to 10 before I am asleep.

Have an "Attitude of Gratitude." I look for something to be grateful for in everything that happens to me. I may not always succeed immediately, but I always succeed eventually. Life is rich; you just have to find and see the bounty in everything.

Get daily fresh air and sunshine. Our natural environment shaped human physiology with ample exposure to sunlight, one of Nature's disease fighters. There are roughly 20,000 genes in our body, and vitamin D affects nearly 3,000 of them, and it also affects vitamin D receptors located throughout the body. Normalize your vitamin D levels with safe amounts of sun exposure. Ten minutes or so in the mid-day sun is good for making this vitamin/hormone. Caucasian sunbathers can get 20,000 IUs in 20 minutes at noon in summer.

Studies:

- A meta-analysis of five studies published in the March 2014 issue of *Anticancer Research* found that patients diagnosed with breast cancer who had high vitamin D levels were twice as likely to survive compared to women with low levels.[40]

- A landmark study reported in 2011 by Creighton University School of Medicine of 1,179 women showed a 60 percent or greater reduction in cancer risk compared to women who did not get the vitamin.[41]

40 Mohr SB, Gorham ED et al. Meta-analysis of Vitamin D Sufficiency for Improving Survival of Patients with Breast Cancer. *Anticancer Research*, March 2014:34(3); 1163-1166

41 Anderson J. The Power of D. http://www.creighton.edu/fileadmin/user/creighton-magazine/archive/PDFs/2007_creightonfall2007.pdf. Creighton University Fall 2007 magazine, p 10-13.

- In animal studies, vitamin D has been found to have several activities that might slow or prevent the development of cancer, including promoting cellular differentiation, decreasing cancer cell growth, stimulating cell death (apoptosis), and reducing tumor blood vessel formation (angiogenesis). It is estimated that 50,000-70,000 Americans die prematurely from various kinds of cancer each year due to insufficient intake of vitamin D.[42]

Research suggests that supplementing between 4,000 IU and 10,000 IU daily promotes good health. Ideally, monitor your vitamin D levels throughout the year.

Control your insulin levels. Eliminate your intake of processed foods and sugars/fructose as much as possible. Never forget that sugar feeds cancer. Carbohydrates such as breads, starches, and starchy vegetables should be eliminated as much as possible also, as they get stored as sugar if they are not immediately burned. Fruit, because it contains fructose, should be severely restricted. Check out the Nourishment Chapter XIII for more information on diet.

Maintain an ideal body weight. We know that if you are overweight or obese, you are at higher risk of developing certain cancers, heart disease, high blood pressure, type 2 diabetes, gallstones, breathing problems, and more. That is why maintaining a healthy weight is so important: It helps you lower your risk for developing these problems, helps you feel good about yourself, and gives you more energy to enjoy life.

But most of all, weight management can help you manage your blood sugar, which is such an important part of the cancer dance. Unfortunately, 95% of diets fail because most people regain their lost weight in 1-5 years.

The problem is that diets are usually focused on counting calories, not on the quality of food and its impact on our hormones. Commercial

---

42 Grant WB, Holick MF. Benefits and requirements of vitamin D for optimal health: a review. *Altern Med Rev.* 2005 Jun; 10(2):94-111.

diet programs also tend to give a thumbs up to zero-calorie sweeteners and the problem there is that we need to retrain our taste buds to not want these sugary-tasting foods. And do we need to mention how wrong the "expert advice" has been on fats? I don't even have a bathroom scale in the house. I don't need it. When you eat whole, organic foods, and balance nutrition with good habits, weight management is not an issue. You just naturally stay more fit.

Build your physical strength. Move your body, which will get your blood flowing and move the lymph. One of the primary reasons exercise works is that it drives your insulin levels down. Controlling insulin levels is one of the most powerful ways to reduce your cancer risks. Your muscles' use of sugar lessens the free-flowing blood sugar. Exercise also builds endorphins, which are anti-cancer. You should try to exercise a minimum of 30 minutes per day. Try walking, yoga, tai chi, and Qigong. Knitting really does create endorphins and is therefore a good anti-cancer exercise. You may have an activity you enjoy—make time for it and move!

Belly breathing. This is one of the most important practices I have learned in my journey. Brenda Stockdale, the Director of Behavioral Medicine, Vantage Oncology/RCOG, taught it to me and the physicians who attended the 2012 Integrative Oncology Conference. She showed case studies of people with cancer who had healed themselves through belly breathing. Dr. David Jockers of Exodus Health Center states:

> Several studies have shown that heart disease, depression, anxiety, and chronic pain patients have an intimate relationship with persistent shallow, chest breathing behaviors. Several researchers have suggested maintenance of posture and breathing habits to be the most important factor in health and energy promotion.

You can read more about the practice of breathing properly and why it is so important here: http://www.naturalhealth365.com/breathing-exercises.html/.

Get good, nourishing sleep every night—at least 7 hours. According to the NIH, an estimated 70 million U.S. adults have chronic sleep or wakefulness disorders. Sleep deficiency can increase the risk of obesity, diabetes, high blood pressure, and other health conditions. Most experts recommend turning off TVs, computers, and other electronic gadgets an hour before bedtime, and they recommend sleeping in a dark room.

These steps help increase the amount of the "anti-cancer hormone" called melatonin our bodies will make each night. Melatonin boosts the immune system and inhibits development of new tumor blood vessels (tumor angiogenesis), which slows the spread of the cancer. It also counteracts estrogen's tendency to stimulate cell growth. But what is the right amount of sleep? The National Sleep Foundation recently issued new Sleep Duration Recommendations. They are:

Age	Recommended	May be appropriate	Not recommended
Newborns *0-3 months*	14 to 17 hours	11 to 13 hours 18 to 19 hours	Less than 11 hours More than 19 hours
Infants *4-11 months*	12 to 15 hours	10 to 11 hours 16 to 18 hours	Less than 10 hours More than 18 hours
Toddlers *1-2 years*	11 to 14 hours	9 to 10 hours 15 to 16 hours	Less than 9 hours More than 16 hours
Preschoolers *3-5 years*	10 to 13 hours	8 to 9 hours 14 hours	Less than 8 hours More than 14 hours
School-aged Children *6-13 years*	9 to 11 hours	7 to 8 hours 12 hours	Less than 7 hours More than 12 hours
Teenagers *14-17 years*	8 to 10 hours	7 hours 11 hours	Less than 7 hours More than 11 hours
Young Adults *18-25 years*	7 to 9 hours	6 hours 10 to 11 hours	Less than 6 hours More than 11 hours
Adults *26-64 years*	7 to 9 hours	6 hours 10 hours	Less than 6 hours More than 10 hours
Older Adults *≥ 65 years*	7 to 8 hours	5 to 6 hours 9 hours	Less than 5 hours More than 9 hours

LIFESTYLE

Court nourishing relationships. The more positive and happy we are, the more our body and our immune system are exposed to the many positive aspects of metabolism. Having loving and supportive relationships helps us feel connected and surrounds us with positive energy. Today's hectic life and the arms-length distance created with social media often make relationships more challenging. Eknath Easwaran writes in his book, *Take Your Time: Finding Balance in a Hurried World,* about the value of patience in our relationships with others:

> Most relationships begin to fall apart through disagreements, and disagreements are not settled by argumentation and logic. They are resolved—or, more accurately, dissolved—through patience. Without patience you start retaliating, and the other person gets more upset and retaliates too. Instead of retaliating with a curt reply, slow down and refrain from answering immediately. As soon as you can manage it, try a smile and a sympathetic word … So much of the richness of life is to be found in companionship that I cannot stress strongly enough how important it is to heal bonds that have weakened and to bring freshness back to relationships that have grown stale.

Have a tool to permanently erase the neurological short-circuiting that can activate cancer genes. Even the CDC states that 85 percent of disease is caused by emotions. It is likely that this factor may be more important than all the other physical ones listed here, so make sure this is addressed.

My particular favorite tool for this purpose is the Emotional Freedom Technique. EFT works on the premise that, no matter what part of life needs improvement, there are unresolved or buried emotional issues in the way. Any kind of emotional stress can hinder the natural healing potential of the body. What I remember from my therapy is that traumas are stored as stagnant energy, so EFT helps move the energy and release the trauma by using a tapping sequence on certain meridian points. Your fingers are used to tap, instead of using needles like in acupuncture.

LIFESTYLE

My experience with EFT was that it was very hard for me to open up those places where I had deeply buried issues that had roots in emotional and psychological trauma; I had a resistance to "going there." I had to keep reminding myself that this was something that nobody could do for me, and that it was perhaps the block to healing the disease. Once I began to open up, it got easier. I found it extremely effective, with a fairly quick response overall.

Reduce your exposure to environmental toxins. We're taking pesticides, household chemical cleaners, scented laundry soaps, synthetic air fresheners, and air pollution. As discussed in Chapter V, many of these materials are endocrine disrupters and/or carcinogenic and are very harmful. You may want to go back and review that section. As patients of cancer and chronic disease, we want to give our bodies and immune systems as much chance to rest as possible.

Reduce your use of cell phones and other wireless technologies. Implement as many safety strategies as possible if/when you cannot avoid their use. As the Breast Cancer Fund states in their research:

> Exposure to non-ionizing radiation in the form of electromagnetic fields (EMF) is linked to many adverse health effects, including breast cancer in both men and women, and is supported by decades of scientific research. One source of continuous daily exposure to EMF is from cell phones in the form of radiofrequency (RF) radiation.
>
> Radiofrequency (RF) radiation, one type of EMF, is continuously emitted from cell phones. A growing body of scientific evidence from around the world supports an association of widespread low-level RF exposure and the negative health outcomes. These include increased risk of breast cancer in both men and women, along with other cancers, Alzheimer's and other neuro-degenerative diseases, reproductive problems, immune function disruption, electrohypersensitivity, and various symptoms such as insomnia, headaches, memory loss, and concentration and attention difficulties.

LIFESTYLE

To minimize exposure, you can use your speakerphone and hold the phone away from you. There are many EMF harmonizing, balancing, and blocking devices on the market. In my experience, some work, some don't. Have I ever bought something that didn't live up to the claims? Sure, but I'll take all the help I can get.

Wow, this is a fun modality! How many times do we get to start over, to redecorate our lives, to renovate and remake ourselves?

I actually changed my name as part of my Healing Platform™. The person I was when I was diagnosed was named Ann, and she was a very serious, intense, driven person who only skimmed the surface of life. So when I changed my life, I changed my name. Annie was my childhood nickname, the name of a fun-loving, adventurous, kind and gentle person.

Be courageous and adventurous in this modality. Find joy and excitement in your choices. Learn how to approve of your choices and your "self."

Welcome to your new life! Let's start by exploring the following:

Is there anything you want to change about yourself or your life? How will you approach this?

_____

_____

_____

_____

_____

Do you have good quality of life? Are you getting sufficient rest, eating well, and laughing regularly? If not, what are your plans to address these issues?

_____

_____

_____

_____

_____

_____

_____

_____

_____

_____

_____

_____

_____

_____

LIFESTYLE

What are you doing for exercise? List your ideas and plans here.

_____

_____

_____

_____

_____

_____

_____

_____

_____

_____

_____

_____

_____

_____

LIFESTYLE

How do you handle stress? What tools are you using or planning on implementing? Create a way to give yourself feedback: marks + or minus, happy or sad on calendar, journal, get feedback from a friend, or use a reminder system to learn what tools are effective.

_____

_____

_____

_____

_____

_____

_____

_____

_____

_____

_____

_____

CHAPTER XVI

Targeted Therapies of Choice

*T*he targeted therapy is stronger because of all the other healing modalities. The first six parts of the Healing Platform heal and strengthen the mind, spirit, immune system, and the vital body organs. The targeted therapy of choice, best-case scenario, is one that will target the cancer, not the person. The body is already weakened or the cancer would not have been able to overpower the immune system.

My main targeted therapy of choice in 2002 was Insulin Potentiation Targeted Low Dose (IPTLD or IPT for short). In July of 2002, about one year after I was diagnosed and given 3-5 months to live, I was still alive but I still had the metastatic disease. I went back to the internet to see what else I could find. In my searches, I read about IPT. I first read about another Stage IV breast cancer patient who went through the treatment with no side-effects and survived. Then I was fascinated to learn that IPT was discovered in 1930 and had been used on cancer since 1946 with a great many successes. Survival story after story convinced me that I was on to something that might work for me. But although the stories were exciting, even more positive was to read about how IPT actually worked.

IPT uses a combination FDA-approved drugs and insulin to target only the cancer cells. Insulin is a biological response modifier. The science shows that diseased cells (cancer in particular) have more insulin receptors on their surfaces than healthy cells.

The IPT therapy protocol calls for the patient to be in a fasting condition. This means that the cancer cells are already hungry and looking for sustenance (sugar). When the healthy cells are deprived of food, they begin to quiet down to conserve energy for the heart, brain, and lungs. The physician administers a small amount of insulin; the dose is formulated to take the patient into a slight hypoglycemic state (low blood sugar) within 25-30 minutes. The insulin further stimulates the cancer cells, so now they are really hungry. Conversely, the hypoglycemic state forces the healthy cells into an even more somnolent (sleepy) posture. Now the physician delivers a fractionated dose—about 10 percent of the conventional dose, which the cancer cells should eagerly receive. The chemo is followed by intravenous medications that are anti-inflammatory, anti-fungal, anti-viral, and anti-bacterial—four things that cancer thrives on. Lastly, a dose of glucose is delivered, which serves to drive the chemo into the cancer cells but will also feed and "wake up" the healthy cells.

My IPT treatments lasted about one hour and were very easy. I sat in a recliner and read until my blood sugar level had fallen to a hypoglycemic state (also called the "therapeutic moment"), then had my treatment, and then drank a Gatorade (provided by the doctor back then) to break my fast.

NOTE: I replaced the Gatorade with healthy shakes and some proteins shortly after starting IPT, because I wanted to use natural sugars and I learned protein would help steady the blood sugar levels.

After treatments, I would go for an ultrasound to see what the tumors were doing, then schedule my next appointment, and then go out for a healthy lunch. I had absolutely no side effects, I never got sick, I never lost my hair. I literally watched all the tumors shrink and disappear. Remember that old CoverGirl ad, "Easy, breezy, CoverGirl"? Well, I felt like the "Easy, breezy, cancer patient."

In conventional oncology, patients are given as big a dose of the chemotherapy drugs as possible, short of outright killing the body's immune system and intestinal tract. The bigger the dose, the more the

THERAPY

drugs can hopefully penetrate the walls of the cancer cell and get inside to kill them. Unfortunately, that much chemo also penetrates healthy cells, especially the rapidly dividing cells like the ones in your intestinal lining, and the ones that grow hair. It's a brutal process with brutal side effects and sometimes even organ failure. As the white blood cell count plummets, the immune system suffers greatly.

IPT is a way to target a small amount of chemo directly to cancer cells. Ever since Otto Warburg won the Nobel Prize in the 1930s, we have known that cancer cells are unique in that they require a lot of sugar (glucose) for their fuel. It is actually the hormone insulin that the body uses to escort sugar into cells, and cancer cells have a lot more *receptors* for insulin—think outstretched hands catching any sugar cubes that pass by in the bloodstream. That need for sugar makes cancer cells vulnerable to whatever you combine with sugar in an IV because cancer cells will take that in, too, as they reach for the sugar.

For example, when you get a PET scan, a radioactive agent is combined with sugar water. The cancer cells scramble to get that sugar and in the process, they also take in the radioactive dye. That produces a picture of your tumor. Now, suppose instead of the dye we add a small amount of the chemo drugs to that sugar water? Yes, it pretty much goes directly to the cancer cells, by-passing the normal cells. It's the Trojan horse concept.

Doctors who administer IPTLD generally use about one-tenth as much chemo and patients generally do not lose their hair, do not experience severe nausea, or most of the side effects known to patients who undergo conventional treatment. IPTLD gets the job done while being much gentler on the body, much kinder to the immune system, and patients have a much better quality of life while going through treatment.

My research told me that doctors who use insulin to target the chemo drugs have a more enlightened approach than those who do not. I felt so good after my IPTLD treatments, I usually spent the rest of my day sightseeing and shopping!

THERAPY

People often ask me, "If IPTLD is so good, why doesn't every doctor's office do it?" Good question. My answer: The use of insulin to "potentiate" or efficiently target drugs into cells is time-honored and time-tested. But, due to lack of clinical trials, it is still considered "experimental" and is not FDA-approved. It is considered an "off-label" use of insulin. Although many drugs are used off label, most physicians do not offer IPTLD as a therapy. I decided to find out when the pharmaceutical companies might run a clinical trial.

After a great many phone calls, I finally reached a pharmaceutical industry executive in 2005 and asked him when they were going to run a clinical trial, since IPTLD had been used successfully on cancer since 1946. He said "never" because they could not justify it on their bottom line. "We are a profitable corporation. We have already tested the chemotherapy drugs. To do it again will cost us millions of dollars, and we stand to lose billions because of the lower dose."

I was not quick enough to say, "But, hey, you stand to win market share because there are so many people who will NOT do conventional therapy because of the side-effects." So, their reasoning is that if the doctors are using one-tenth as much chemo and getting better outcomes, that cuts into sales. I think the situation amounts to a very unfortunate lost opportunity for consumers—people like you and me.

I persist in being optimistic, however. I know that the way to getting IPT some visibility and better mainstream acceptance is through statistics and studies. Since the pharmaceutical companies will not pay for these, Best Answer for Cancer Foundation (BAFC) has decided to take the road-less-traveled: the difficult one of self-funded studies. In 2010, BAFC received approval from Liberty Institutional Review Board (IRB) for a study titled "A Quality of Life Study Using Insulin Potentiation Targeted Low Dose (IPTLD^{SM}) Chemotherapy and Nutrition Therapy in the Treatment of Cancer." The study will measure the quality-of-life of cancer patients undergoing targeted low dose chemo instead of conventional chemo. We believe that the results of this study will show a much more favorable outcome than similar studies for conventional chemotherapy.

THERAPY

That was the first IRB-sanctioned study of IPT in the United States. In 2015, BAFC received approval for the study "The IPTLD Survival Outcomes Study for Stage IV Cancer Patients Using CST and IV Therapies." The purpose of this study will be to treat Stage IV cancer patients with an IPTLD integrative protocol and measure their survival outcomes. The study mimics that of Dr. James Forsythe, an integrative oncologist from Reno, Nevada, (http://www.drforsythe.com) whose five-year overall survival rate for adult Stage IV cancers is 67%, a phenomenal result compared to conventional cancer care.

Patients interested in joining this study should contact Best Answer for Cancer Foundation at admin@bestanswerforcancer.org.

Other targeted cancer therapies/substances (many not made or promoted by pharmaceutical companies) are:

• **High-dose IV Vitamin C**

High-dose vitamin C has been studied as a treatment for patients with cancer since the 1970s. It works by creating hydrogen peroxide, which damages the DNA and mitochondria of cancer cells, shuts down their energy supply, and kills them. Vitamin C is "selectively toxic" meaning it does not harm healthy cells. Also, cancer does not build resistance to vitamin C as it will to chemotherapy, and the therapy has little or no side-effects. High-dose vitamin C may be given intravenously; some clinics will start at 35 grams and work up according to tolerance.

It is worth noting that the infamous "Moertel study" done in the mid-1980s found no benefit in using vitamin C with cancer.[43] However, that study used a comparatively low dose of *oral* vitamin C that had to navigate the digestive system which greatly limited its absorption. At oral doses above 1 gram per day, absorption in the gut falls to

---

43 Moertel CG, Fleming TR, Creagan ET, Rubin J, O'Connell MJ, Ames MM. High-dose vitamin C versus placebo in the treatment of patients with advanced cancer who have had no prior chemotherapy. A randomized double-blind comparison. *N Engl J Med* 1985;312:137-41.

less than 50 percent and the rest is excreted in the urine.[44] Later studies found that when vitamin C is given intravenously, it does indeed reach levels at which it kills cancer cells.[45] The most recent studies will perhaps turn the tables again. The new liposomal delivery system, where oral vitamin C is encapsulated in fat to slide right through the gut wall, is said to able to deliver levels almost as high as the IV delivery system.[46]

Why some doctors still quote the "highly flawed" Moertel study to dissuade people from IV vitamin C therapy is beyond me. To me, vitamin C is a no brainer. But perhaps it is a case of not following up on newer journals or of following the money. Cancer is a multi-billion-dollar industry, and the pharmaceutical companies are the primary beneficiaries. Since chemotherapy is a revenue-generating drug, it stands to reason that it would be the primary focus of studies, funding, and marketing.

- **Targeted Treatments for Cancer Stem Cells (CSCs)**

Max Wicha, M.D., told us that standard cancer treatments can make things worse because when tumor cells die under assault from chemotherapy and radiation, they give off inflammatory messengers that can recruit cancer stem cells (CSCs).[47,48] CSCs used to be a radical idea. Then in 2012, three studies on the existence of CSCs were published simultaneously in the journals *Nature* and *Science*. Now they have been proven to exist and further study has shown their importance.

---

44 NIH Vitamin C Fact Sheet for Professionals, https://ods.od.nih.gov/factsheets/VitaminC-HealthProfessional

45 Li Y, Schellhorn HE. New Developments and Novel Therapeutic Perspectives for Vitamin C. J. Nutr. October 2007;137:2171-2184

46 Hickey S, Roberts H. Vitamin C and Cancer: Is There A Use For Oral Vitamin C? *Journal of Orthomolecular Medicine*, Vol 28, No 1, 2013

47 Wicha MS, Liu S, and Dontu G. Cancer Stem Cells: An Old Idea—A Paradigm Shift. *Cancer Res* 2006; 66: (4). February 15, 2006 http://www.health.harvard.edu/flu-resource-center/how-to-boost-your-immune-system.htm

48 Bowman BM, Wicha MS. Cancer Stem Cells: A Step Toward the Cure. *JCO* June 10, 2008 vol. 26 no. 17 2795-2799

THERAPY

CSCs are partially responsible for the recurrence of cancer and for the fact metastatic cancer is so difficult to treat—and that is where the majority of deaths come from, so targeting the cancer stem cell population is essential for improving outcomes.[49,50,51] Chemo and radiation do not kill CSCs; conventional therapy actually stimulates metastases. The body can think the dying cancer cells need to be replaced and CSCs can do that. Targeted therapies can tell these stem cells *not* to replace the dying cancer cells.

Targeted treatment for CSCs include metformin, berberine, natural botanicals,[52] curcumin,[53,54] fermented soy, fish oil,[55] modified citrus pectin (PectaSol-C), Heparin, and sulforaphane (found in cruciferous vegetables such as cabbage and broccoli).[56] They actually kill the stem cells.

Caffeine may be able to go hand-in-hand with these targeted stem cell therapies, in that it appears to prevent cancer cells from repairing

49 Hill RP, Milas L. The proportion of stem cells in murine tumors. *Int J Radiat Oncol Biol Phys.* Feb 1989;16(2):513–8

50 West CM, Davidson SE, Hunter RD. Evaluation of surviving fraction at 2 Gy as a potential prognostic factor for the radiotherapy of carcinoma of the cervix. *Int J Radiat Biol.* 1989;56:761–5

51 Diehn M, Cho RW, Clarke MF. Therapeutic Implications of the Cancer Stem Cell Hypothesis. *Semin Radiat Oncol.* 2009 April; 19(2):78-86

52 Fu B, Xue J et al. Chrysin inhibits expression of hypoxia-inducible factor-1α through reducing hypoxia-inducible factor-1α stability and inhibiting its protein synthesis, *Mol Cancer Ther.* January 2007 6; 220-06

53 Subramaniam D, Ramalingam S, Houchen CW, Anant S. Cancer stem cells: a novel paradigm for cancer prevention and treatment. *Mini Rev Med Chem.* 2010 May;10(5):359-71.

54 Kakarala M, Brenner DE, Korkaya H et al. Targeting breast stem cells with the cancer preventive compounds curcumin and piperine. *Breast Cancer Res Treat.* 2010 Aug;122(3):777-85.

55 Hegde S, Kaushal N et al. Δ12-prostaglandin J3, an omega-3 fatty acid–derived metabolite, selectively ablates leukemia stem cells in mice. *Blood.* December 22, 2011 vol. 118 no. 26 6909-6919

56 Rakesh K Srivastava, Su-Ni Tang et al. *Front Biosci* (Elite Ed). 2011 ;3:515-28. Epub 2011 Jan 1

THERAPY

themselves. I envision the day when stronger therapies for cancer stem cells will be available in clinics.

- **Oxidative Therapies**

Ozone therapy (O3)—It is because of my training as an Indoor Air Quality (IAQ) Consultant that I know that ozone is oxygen gas with one extra O molecule (O_3). It is what makes our sky blue. This extra molecule will split off and merge with other molecules to convert them to a substance that is safe for humans. It is because of this quality that we are able to live on this planet: ozone controls the viruses, fungus, and bacteria in our environment by converting them to harmless substances. Used intravenously, it inactivates bacteria, viruses, fungi, yeast and protozoa in our bodies, and it boosts the immune system.

According to Dr. David Minkoff (www.lifeworkswellnesscenter.com):

"Cancer tissue does not do well with oxygen, and mitochondria in cancer tissue do not process oxygen correctly in order to make ATP. We use ozone to remedy this. It improves immune function, oxygen utilization, and with that survival."

Dr. Robert Rowen, who has been treating cancer and chronic disease with many different ozone therapies for 20 years, taught doctors in Sierra Leone in 2015 to use the therapy for Ebola with success. (http://www.docrowen.com/ozone-therapy.html).

Hydrogen peroxide (H2O2)—Uses the same free radical killing mechanism that the immune system uses to eradicate foreign invaders. Cells make hydrogen peroxide to generate free radicals to kill errant cells, viruses, and bacteria. "Hydrogen peroxide is cheaper for the patient, easier for the staff, and more user friendly than ozone in that a smaller needle can be used," according to James Forsythe, M.D., H.M.D., of Nevada (http://www.drforsythe.com).

Prolozone®—This is a homeopathic/oxygen injection technique for all forms of musculo-skeletal and joint pain including chronic neck and back pain, rotator cuff injuries, degenerative and arthritic hips and knees, degenerated discs, and shoulder and elbow pain. The technique was developed by Dr. Frank Shallenberger of the Nevada Clinic in Carson City, NV. He has trained many other physicians worldwide in this technique.

Ultraviolet Therapy—Nature uses the sun's ultraviolet (UV) energy to cleanse the earth. UV light is now used as a disinfectant in hospitals, laboratories, water purification plants, commercial buildings, and food processing plants. UV light is also used to clean blood for hospital transfusions because it is the only known system that cleans blood thoroughly of bacteria and viruses. UV is a well-accepted therapy wherein a portion of blood is drawn from the patient and exposed to cleansing ultraviolet light and then reinfused into the patient's body. This helps the immune system by eliminating viruses and bacteria. It also appears to activate immune system white blood cells, help with blood viscosity (thin out thick, sticky blood), and increase the ability of the blood to carry oxygen.

Ultraviolet Blood Irradiation (UBI) is the same procedure as UV with one addition: Ozone is added to the blood prior to reinfusing it back into the patient's body. Tom Lowe, President of DrsUBI (www.DrsUBI. com) and the Society of Oxidative and Photonic Medicine (www. SOPmed.com) says, "UBI therapy has been overlooked for decades as a viable cancer treatment—a terrible loss for millions of patients who could benefit. It's also a quick, drug-free cure for most infections, even serious ones like polio." Mr. Lowe sells UBI machines to medical professionals; I have an ozone generator from him for home use.

Hyperbaric Oxygen Therapy (HBOT)—This is the use of high pressure oxygen as a drug to treat basic pathophysiologic processes and their diseases. You've probably seen scuba divers use an HBOT chamber to normalize their blood after decompression. In a hyperbaric oxygen therapy chamber, the air pressure is increased several times higher than normal air pressure. This enables your lungs to gather more oxygen than would be possible breathing pure oxygen at normal air pressure. Your blood then carries this oxygen throughout the body which helps fight bacteria and stimulate the release of growth factors and stem cells that promote healing.

THERAPY

In 2013, an animal study on the ketogenic diet combined with hyperbaric oxygen therapy at China Medical University in Taiwan concluded that the two "produce significant anti-cancer effects when combined in a natural model of systemic metastatic cancer. Our evidence suggests that these therapies should be further investigated as potential non-toxic treatments or adjuvant therapies to standard care for patients with systemic metastatic disease."[57]

- **Thermal Medicine: Hyperthermia & Focused Hyperthermia**

Thermal medicine is the manipulation of body or tissue temperature for the treatment of disease. Cultures from around the world can point to ancient uses of hot and cold therapy for medical applications, including cancer. Modern research in thermal medicine aims to understand molecular, cellular, and physiological effects of temperature manipulation and the "stress" response.

Hyperthermia is clinically used for cancer treatment, particularly in combination with radiation and chemotherapy. The idea is that by heating the tumor, it potentiates the chemo and radiation. There are different techniques—everything from "whole body" hyperthermia where they put you under anesthesia, to focused hyperthermia where just the tumor is targeted. In the summer of 2015, I visited the Center for Thermal Oncology in Santa Monica, CA, and met with Drs. Oscar Streeter and Sean Devlin. I underwent targeted hyperthermia and fractionated chemotherapy as a sort of "tune up." It was painless with no side effects and was actually fairly comfortable. Read more at http://www.i2med.com.

THERAPY

---

57 Poff AM, Ari C et al. The Ketogenic Diet and Hyperbaric Oxygen Therapy Prolong Survival in Mice with Systemic Metastatic Cancer. *PLoS ONE*, 2013;8(6): e65522. doi:10.1371/journal.pone.0065522

- **Baking Soda IV Therapy (Sodium Bicarbonate (NaHCO3)**

Pioneered by an oncologist in Italy, Dr. Tullio Simoncini, intravenous baking soda therapy is based on his treatment of cancer as a fungus. He says that sodium bicarbonate, unlike other anti-fungal remedies to which the fungus can become immune, is able to penetrate the tumor and disintegrate it. This speed at which this happens makes fungi's adaptability impossible, rendering it defenseless.

Dr. Simoncini likes to get the sodium bicarbonate as close to the involved organ as possible by "using oral administration for the digestive tract, enemas for the rectum, douching for the vagina and uterus, intravenous injection for the lung and the brain, and inhalation for the upper airways. Breasts, lymph nodes, and subcutaneous lumps can be treated with local injections. The internal organs can be treated locating suitable catheters in the arteries (of the liver, pancreas, prostate, and limbs) or in the cavities of the pleura or peritoneum." There are many physicians in around the world who deliver intravenous baking soda therapy.

A cancer patient named Jim Kelmun, who cured his own cancer with this, developed a home remedy version. It is based on creating an alkaline environment in the body and in the cancer cells. It is a combination of apple cider vinegar, sodium bicarbonate (use only aluminum-free baking soda), and Grade B maple syrup (to encourage the mixture to enter the cancer cells). You can find details on the recipe and the do's and don'ts here: http://www.life-saving-naturalcures-and-naturalremedies.com/natural-cancer-cures-baking-soda-maple-syrup-treatment.html.

- **IV Chelation**

This is an intravenous therapy, usually done in a series of 30 or more. It uses EDTA, a synthetic amino acid that forms a tight chemical bond with lead, cadmium, and other metals and carries them out of the body in the urine. The idea here is that stored heavy metals are inflammatory and interact with pathogens in building biofilm and other defenses to hide from the immune system. Chronic, whole body (systemic) inflammation is now recognized to be behind just about every chronic illness, including cancer. Chelation got FDA approval in 1948 to get

THERAPY

the lead out of sailors who were inundated with it while painting battleships and docks with lead-based paint. It turned out that sailors who also had heart disease saw unexpected improvements in angina and circulation. That's when its anti-inflammatory effects were found. There is no disputing that heavy metals are extremely toxic. The human body is engineered to remove small amounts daily, but not the large amounts we often pick up from modern sources. Chelation became embroiled in controversy—EDTA is not a patentable pharmaceutical—but it is very much available and of great benefit to almost everyone who uses it. It addresses the body's toxic overload.

• **Immunotherapies**

Conventional onocology is coming around to the idea that the immune system can be used to fight cancer. This is generally done by stimulating your immune system with drugs to work harder or smarter to attack cancer cells, or by giving you immune system components, such as genetically modified viruses or modified T-cells to kill cancer cells. It's a growing field. Intergrative oncologists have long made use of a number of complementary therapies to mediate the immune system slowly and safely; the drugs do it faster and with more risk and more side effects (and probably with considerably more expense). But if you have a stage IV cancer, then you may decide it is worth the risk.

"Over the past decade there has been an abundance of basic science and clinic research done by pharmaceutical companies that has evaluated how the immune system handles cancer and have, in the process, developed numerous immune based therapies," said Dr. Sean Devlin (http://www.i2med.com). "With the advent and clinical success of checkpoint inhibitors as well as some cancer vaccines, there has been a wellspring of data to suggest we are entering a new paradigm in the field of oncology. The new found excitement around immunotherapy comes from the fact that it is one treatment approach that holds the promise of a life-long cure."

There are a variety of immunotherapy agents being used now— former President Jimmy Carter was treated in 2015 with a checkpoint inhibitor, for example—and even more coming down the pipeline.

THERAPY

- **RIGVIR® Virotherapy**

This is a prescription virotherapy agent, the first to come to market and the only one that is not genetically modified. The drug contains a live virus that seeks out and selectively infects tumor cells. Once inside, the virus destroys the cancer cell. Healthy cells are not affected, resulting in no side effects and a high quality of life. There is clinical experience of RIGVIR in the treatment of melanoma, stomach cancer, colorectal cancer, pancreatic cancer, kidney cancer, uterine cancer, bladder cancer, lung cancer, prostate cancer and several types of sarcomas.

RIGVIR was developed in Europe and is readily available in the Baltic states of Latvia and Georgia. In the United States, it is not FDA-approved, so it must be obtained by traveling to Latvia and Georgia, or Mexico where Dr. Tony Jimenez also uses RIGVIR. (www.hope4cancer.com). He says, "RIGVIR is supported by a legacy of over 50 years of research that includes numerous clinical trials and it has an exceptional safety profile."

- **Enzymatic Therapy**

Enzymes are considered the "labor force" in living things. Vitamins and minerals are building blocks; enzymes are the busy worker bees. They are the catalysts that initiate, speed up, slow down, or stop biochemical processes. There are three kinds of enzymes: enzymes inherent in raw foods to help us digest them; digestive enzymes secreted by the salivary glands, stomach, pancreas, small intestine, liver, and gall bladder to digest food; and systemic enzymes produced by the body for critical metabolic functions such as immunity, blood and body fluid cleansing and filtering, cell reproduction.

Digestive enzymes. Cancer patients typically have issues with digestion and absorption, plus the standard American diet contains almost no raw food and that tends to deplete our digestive enzymes as we get older. When food is heated more than 116 degrees, all enzymes are killed. If we don't consume a lot of raw food, our body has to donate systemic enzymes meant to do other jobs. Almost none of the foods we eat could be absorbed into our bloodstream without the action of enzymes

THERAPY

working to break down food to extract vital nutrients. Without this break down, undigested food passes into the colon, where it can lead to bloating, gas, diarrhea, cramping, and eventually trigger food allergies and autoimmune diseases. Supplemental digestive enzymes can be very useful. There are some different options out there. Pepsin, papaya, bromelain, and trypsin, for example, break down only proteins and work best in temperatures above our own body temperature of 98.6. I think a better choice for digestive enzymes are the broad spectrum supplemental plant enzymes that break down proteins, fats, carbohydrates, fiber, starches, dairy, and sugar. Plant enzyme supplements such as Integrative Therapeutics' Similase® work roughly in a pH range of 3.0 to 9.0 which covers the variations of gastrointestinal pH conditions.

Systemic enzymes. These give the body the capacity to do work—to heal, reproduce, make new tissue. Proteolytic, or protein-eating enzymes, when taken on an empty stomach, will start cleaning house by cleaning the blood and eating away at fibrin that contributes to inflammation. Systemic enzymes will eat away at the fibrous protein coating that cancer cells and viruses use to cloak themselves from the immune system. Enzymes also help with a most important issue for cancer patients—quality of life. Clinical studies reported in 2008 demonstrated that "systemic enzyme therapy significantly decreased tumor-induced and therapy-induced side effects and complaints such as nausea, gastrointestinal complaints, fatigue, weight loss, and restlessness and obviously stabilized the quality of life."[58] The idea behind systemic enzyme therapy is that enzymes inhibit rapidly dividing cells, a hallmark of cancer.

Our understanding of this started in the early 1900s when Scottish embryologist John Beard noted that a human fetus starts with one cell and multiplies rapidly into all kinds of different cells—heart, lung, bone, eyes—but at some point, the process shifts to where cells replicate only as more of the same kind. Dr. Beard noticed that on the 56th

---

58 Beuth J. Proteolytic enzyme therapy in evidence-based complementary oncology: fact or fiction? *Integr Cancer Ther*, 2008 Dec;7(4):311-6

day of gestation, the fetal pancreas starts producing enzymes, which stopped this rapid growth of undifferentiated cells.

Fast forward to the 1960s when Dr. William D. Kelley was diagnosed with pancreatic cancer, and he used Beard's philosophy to develop his own therapy using diet, enzymes, colonics and a program that addressed his life on multiple levels. He then began successfully treating cancer patients. To this day, his patients still number among the decades-long survivors of pancreatic and difficult cancers. I particularly like his approach because it validates mine, in part: you look at the whole being, not just the cancer. You can read about Dr. Kelley and his protocol here: http://www.drkelley.info/.

In the 1980s, Dr. Nicholas Gonzalez of New York conducted a formal study of Kelley's work and subsequently became a leader in the modern use of enzymes, along with diet and detoxification therapies as a primary treatment for major cancers. He had hundreds of patients with pancreatic and other cancers living at least five years after being told they didn't have much time left. He convinced the National Cancer Institute in 1998 to fund a clinical trial to compare his enzyme-nutritional therapy with the best chemotherapy available for the treatment of advanced pancreatic cancer. Some called the effort the most significant investigation of an unconventional cancer treatment to date sanctioned by the federal government, driven by consumer demand for less toxic treatments and better outcomes. How did it turn out? Well, in 2012 Dr. Gonzalez wrote the book, *What Went Wrong: The Truth Behind the Clinical Trial of the Enzyme Treatment of Cancer,* that documents why he felt the government sabotaged the trial.

As we get older and have eaten a lifetime of the standard American diet, our enzymes levels are depleted because we eat mostly processed and cooked food which contains no living enzymes. Systemic enzymes are measured in Units of Fibrolytic Activity, meaning how much fibrin they break down in a set amount of time. Different formulations target different activity in the body:

THERAPY

- Nattokinase is made from the traditional Japanese food called natto which is the fermented form of boiled soybeans. It is said to have similar clot-dissolving abilities as plasmin, an enzyme that we all have in our blood as our natural defense mechanism to dissolve unwanted blood clots. The body's coagulation system is a complicated and highly regulated system. Modern lifestyles often tip the balance toward hypercoagulation (thick blood). Over a prolonged period of time, the tissues of the body gradually become hypoxic (lacking oxygen) and the internal environment becomes acidic. That's an invitation to cancer and other chronic diseases. The human body produces several types of enzymes for making blood clot (thrombus), but only one main enzyme for breaking it down and dissolving it—plasmin. Blood clots form when strands of protein called fibrin accumulate in a blood vessel. Thrombolytic enzymes are naturally generated in the lining (endothelial cells) of the blood vessels. As the body ages, production of these enzymes begins to decline, making blood more prone to coagulation. This can contribute to dementia, heart disease, and cancer. Nattokinase is considered a better and safer option than aspirin and pharmaceutical blood thinners.

- Lumbrokinase is made from earthworms. It is another enzyme source that addresses hypercoagulation. At our annual conferences, I've invited Canada RNA who makes the product known as Boluoke because, according to the company, it is "the only lumbrokinase that has been thoroughly researched and its enzymatic strength standardized. Other lumbrokinase products currently on the market may cite Boluoke's credentials and research, but are not disclosing the enzymatic strength of their lumbrokinase. Research has shown that 40mg lumbrokinase, is much more potent 720mg nattokinase."

- Serrapeptase is made from a microorganism in silkworm, and has been used clinically for over 30 years throughout Europe and Asia with none of the dangerous side effects of NSAIDS. It has been used in the United States since 1997. This is a proteolytic, fibrin-eating, anti-inflammatory enzyme. Dr. Hans Nieper, the German physician who pioneered the use of serrapeptase, said, "Unlike other biological enzymes, serrapeptase affects only non-living tissue … Serrapeptase dissolves only dead tissues such as the old fibrous layers that clog the lining of our arteries and dangerously restrict the flow of blood and oxygen to the brain. Serrapeptase digests all non-living tissue, cysts, blood clots, inflammation, and arterial blockages."[59] It is reported to be more effective than the use of EDTA chelation for removing arterial plaque; EDTA pulls out heavy metals, but serrapeptase actually "eats away" at the plaque. Serrapeptase has been used for the treatment of cardiovascular problems, varicose veins, pain, arthritis, fibrocystic breast disease, lung problems, carpal tunnel syndrome, and sports injuries. It is thought to thin the fluids formed from inflammation or injury and facilitates their drainage which speeds the tissue repair process. World Nutrition makes a serrapeptase product called Vitälzȳm. It is a powerful enzyme, best taken in small doses.

• Wobenzyme was introduced in Germany in 1960. It is a broad-spectrum blend of plant-based enzymes that has shown the ability to fight cancer because it reduces systemic inflammation. There are four different versions of this product: Wobenzym, Wobenzym Plus (classic), Wobenzym N, and Wobenzym PS (Professional Strength). According to Dr. Juergen Winkler (www.qfmed.com), "Wobenzym N has six ingredients: Papain, bromelian, rutoside, trypsin, chymotrypsin and pancreatic. While the Wobenzym PS and Plus contain only rutoside, trypsin and bromelian. Wobenzym N has additional ingredients and is reportedly more helpful for immune system function. The Wobenzym N is more comprehensive and given my studies on enzymes and cancer, it appears this

---

59 Nieper HA. Accessed at http://www.agriorganics.com/natural.php?Pid=46

formula is more comprehensive for cancer, immune dysfunction and inflammation." I take Wobenzym N for my immune system.

"Enzymes are simple, powerful, yet often forgotten," said Donese Worden, NMD, (www.drworden.com). "Sometimes we are so busy looking at the glitzy new therapies, we overlook the basics and enzymes are very efficient tools for cancer. For starters, using enzymes means we help the patient to make more energy (ATP) with less effort."

- **Colonic Therapy**

Digestive problems are all around us, and the colon "takes a hit." Bacteria, yeast, and parasites can live in a polluted environment in the colon and that can become one more thing overloading the immune system. During a colonic, the colon's walls constantly get flushed with purified water that removes mucous and hardened fecal matter where bacteria, parasites, and Candida albicans-filled pockets can be hiding out. The idea of rinsing the large intestine and the rectum is to take away a pathogen's source of nourishment. It's a safe, simple, time-honored method of detoxification. Adding coffee to the colonic therapy can also help detoxify the liver and the gallbladder.

Using colonics for healing purposes has been around for ages. The pharaohs of Egypt had their "guardians of the anus," a doctor who specialized in administering the enemas and keeping bowels clean. In the 1700s, enemas were a common practice in France, considered indispensable for vibrant health. This therapy has fallen out of favor with today's medical establishment, but it is quite effective. Until about 1984, the coffee enema procedure was listed in the *Merck Manual*, a handbook for physicians. Dr. Max Gerson (1881-1959) introduced coffee colonics into cancer therapy in the 1930s. Based on German laboratory work, Gerson believed that caffeine could stimulate the liver and gall bladder to discharge bile, contributing to the health of the cancer patient. Although coffee can be irritating to the stomach, coffee provides certain phytochemicals, specifically kahweol and cafestol. These nutrients activate glutathione, which is a primary antioxidant.

An enema cleanses just the last six inches or so of the large intestine called the rectum; a colonic goes roughly 15 inches higher up the large intestine. An enema is good for constipation, but the more thorough colonic is for detoxification. Most colonic therapists undergo a training process that leads to certification.

I think of colonics as fascinating "BM-TV" (pun intended). Many of the machines have a well-lighted tube where you can see what comes out—gas, mucus, bile... One time I saw green beans, perfectly shaped beans, come out. I guess I wasn't chewing my food.

- **Medical Cannabis**

This is not the marijuana of the hippy generation. Originally, marijuana plants were a balanced combination of two key compounds, THC and CBD. But growers bred out the CBD because it didn't contribute to the "high." Both compounds have benefits for cancer, and have different physical and emotional effects. CBD is less euphoric; people report their brains feel sharper and they have more energy. There are different combinations of THC and CBD for each disease/issue. For example, medical cannabis formulations that are high in THC are not recommended for an ER-positive breast cancer patient because high THC apparently can foster more cancer cell growth. Eloise Thiesen, a registered nurse, is my go-to source. She consults with United Patients Group, a 501(c)3 nonprofit dedicated to educating and raising awareness about medical cannabis. (http://unitedpatientsgroup.com). Beware of random internet sources for cannabis because you don't know what you're getting and the material often is not certified for purity. Get a consult with a professional.

- **Zolodex Injections (stops ovaries' Estrogen production)**

Zolodex (goserelin) is an allopathic, prescription hormone therapy drug used for estrogen positive (ER+) breast cancer as well as prostate cancers. In breast cancer, its function is to shut down the estrogen production of the ovaries. I learned about this therapy from my second opinion physician at the University of Texas Health Science Center in

THERAPY

San Antonio. I remember him turning to my then-husband after I had received the injection and saying, "Okay, prepare yourself. Your wife has just entered menopause. You can expect hot flashes, night sweats, and irritability." Fortunately, I had only the hot flashes, but it seemed a small price to pay to stop feeding the cancer.

Zolodex is an injection in the belly fat that can be delivered monthly or every three months. The size of the needle is huge (and scary!) and, without numbing the belly with ice or a medication, can be quite painful. For this reason and to lessen the number of doctor visits, I chose to have the injection every three months.

I don't know of any natural substances that will do what this drug does. In retrospect, I would do it again; mind you, I was at an age where preserving the option to have children was not important.

- **Femara/Arimidex (Aromatase inhibitor)**

My second opinion physician also recommended an aromatase inhibitor. He told me that when the ovaries stop producing estrogen, the adrenals get helpful and start creating an estrogen-like enzyme called aromatase which turns the hormone androgen into small amounts of estrogen in the body. In order to more completely starve the cancer, I would need to take an aromatase inhibitor. There are a few out there: Arimidex®, Aromase®, and Femara®. I settled on Femara because it seemed to have the fewest side effects and it was the cheapest. It comes in pill form, and it is taken daily. I have recently learned of natural substances that are aromatase inhibitors such as melatonin, nettles (Mediherb tincture), frankincense, and resveratrol. I am currently looking into dosages and costs with the intention of switching over.

- **Poly-MVA®**

When you bind alpha lipoic acid and vitamin B1 to the trace mineral palladium by way of an electrical charge, you have a dietary supplement called Poly-MVA. It is a popular cancer tool with IOICP physicians because it enhances and protects the process of making energy (ATP) properly in the mitochondria (energy factories in each one of our cells).

In other words, it gets at the heart of accurate cell replication, helping cells have enough energy to replicate properly. Poly-MVA can be taken orally and intravenously. Read about it at http://www.polymva.com.

Dr. James Forsythe (http://www.drforsythe.com) ran a study in 2004-2006 of 225 cancer patients where he treated cancer with Poly-MVA alone, and with Poly-MVA combined with chemotherapy. His overall survival rate on the combined therapy was 32 percent, which was much better than standard chemotherapy alone. In 2010, Dr. Forsythe began studying the survival outcomes of Poly-MVA delivered in a program called Forsythe Immune Protocol (FIP) into which he added the therapies IPT-Lite, L-glutathione, IV vitamin C, and a modified Myers Cocktail. He is reporting a 71 percent survival rate after six years! Best Answer for Cancer Foundation is duplicating this study under the oversight of an Institutional Review Board (IRB). There are several physicians in the United States who are participating in this study. If you are interested in joining the study, please write admin@bestanswerforcancer.org.

- **Lugol's Iodine Solution**

Most cancer patients are iodine deficient. Dr. David Derry who wrote the book, *Breast Cancer and Iodine*, proposed that iodine and thyroid hormone work as an anti-cancer team. Iodine, he said, is the primary trigger for natural cell death (apoptosis) and the main surveillance mechanism for abnormal cells. He said iodine is "by far the best antibiotic, antiviral and antiseptic of all time." Iodine is able to penetrate quickly through the cell walls of single-celled microorganisms, no matter their defenses. Dr. Derry felt that if American women had sufficient levels of iodine and thyroid hormone, breast cancer would just about disappear. Iodized salt does not provide enough iodine to meet the body's needs. But one drop per day of Lugol's (a combination of iodine and potassium iodide) can do that, he said. The use of iodine often goes hand-in-hand with natural thyroid hormone supplementation. To learn more: http://www.westonaprice.org/modern-diseases/the-great-iodine-debate.

THERAPY

Lugol's is also a very handy antiseptic to keep in the medicine cabinet for mosquito bites, bee stings, and also to treat scars, moles, and those odd barnacle-like things that sometimes pop up on our skin. It tends to stay in that local area for several days, combating pathogens. Some doctors tell women to "paint their breasts" periodically with iodine because it protects the mammary glands.

- **Curcumin**

Curcumin is the active principal ingredient in the herb turmeric that is used liberally in Indian cuisine. It is an anti-inflammatory, anti-oxidant, anti-microbial, and anti-carcinogenic herb. It is probably the most researched botanical, with more than 5,000 peer-reviewed studies on it. It is used to prevent and treat cancers and other chronic diseases. Although pharmaceutical inhibitors of cyclooxygenase-2 (COX-2), HER2, tumor necrosis factor (TNF), EGFR, and vascular endothelial cell growth factor (VEGF) have been approved for human use by the FDA, curcumin as a single agent can down-regulate all these targets and more. Curcumin also inhibits growth and renewal of tumor stem cells.[60],[61] Dr. Ajay Goel of Baylor University Medical Center in Dallas, TX, one of the leading researchers of it, said there is evidence curcumin impacts epigenetic pathways that play a pivotal and frequent role in most human diseases, including cancers. In other words, having about 250 mg a day of curcumin in our diet or as a supplement encourages our genes to express in good ways, not bad. It comes in liposomal form. Remember, most cancers are greatly influenced by dietary and environmental factors.

According to Dr. Winkler, the intravenous form is best. "Curcumin, a turmeric derivative, can be taken orally but alone is poorly

60 Subramaniam D, Ramalingam S et al. Cancer stem cells: a novel paradigm for cancer prevention and treatment. *Mini Rev Med Chem.* 2010 May;10(5):359-71.

61 Kakarala M, Brenner DE et al. Targeting breast stem cells with the cancer preventive compounds curcumin and piperine. *Breast Cancer Res Treat.* 2010 Aug;122(3):777-85.

absorbed by the body. It requires fat or oil to aid in absorption along with pepper. There are several new liposomal formulations which may aid in it absorption and utilization by the body. In my opinion the best way to get most things into the body at controlled concentration is to give it intravenously. Intravenous forms of curcumin go directly into the body and we know how much we have given and it does not require first being absorbed by the GI tract and then going through the liver where it might be changed or passed out of the body."

Not many U.S. doctors seem to making use of IV curcumin these days. However, I have had curcumin via IV during IPT instead of chemo, and I felt a real biological response. I got very warm and flushed; it was quite different from the way my IPT treatments usually felt.

- **Metformin and Berberine**

In 2005, researchers in Scotland found unexpectedly low rates of cancer among diabetics taking metformin. Follow-up studies reported as much as a 50 percent reduction in risk. Exposure to metformin reduces the cellular mutation rate and the accumulation of DNA damage. Metformin may be the safest prescription drug for diabetes, but research shows the herbal supplement berberine can lower blood sugar as well as metformin.[62] Berberine is a powerful botanical revered in Chinese and Ayurvedic medicine. Research shows it also has the ability to lower triglycerides and blood pressure, to fight infections, and boost intestinal health. Animal research suggests it inhibits the growth of cancer cells. Both metformin and berberine exert a positive influence on cancer stem cells and metastases. They are inexpensive and I take both.

- **Haelan 951**

This is a non-GMO fermented soy medical food-type liquid supplement with multi-modial properties. According to the company, it "provides the ideal nutritional support for cancer patients suffering from cachexia, anorexia, protein calorie malnutrition, the toxic side

62 Yin J et al. Efficacy of berberine in patients with type 2diabetes mellitus. *Metabolism.* 2008 May; 57 (5):712-717

effects of chemotherapy, and undesirable hormonal imbalances that promote faster tumor growth. Hormonal imbalances are managed by decreasing estrogen receptor-alpha (ER-a) sites, increasing estrogen receptor-beta (ER-b) sites, increased cellular immunity by increasing 2-methoxy-estradiol and other compounds that have an affinity for the estrogen receptor-beta sites. In addition, other properties of this nutritional support reduces NF-Kb, increases P-21 cellular levels (via the P-53 pathway) anti-angiogenesis and anti-inflammatory cytokine immune responses while simultaneously increasing immune cytokine responses that induce stem cell differentiation."

The key here is whether soy is impacting the alpha or the beta estrogen receptors. We know that about 90 of breast cancers are driven by estrogen that goes to the alpha receptors. Unfermented soy goes to the alpha receptor sites and unhealthy people have a higher amount of alpha receptor sites. Haelan 951's soy is fermented, meaning the process has broken down the estrogen in the soy so the body does not have to process it. Haelan also increases the number of beta receptors so it lowers the amount of circulating estrogen in the body.[63] The National Institutes of Health studied the product and reported in 2015 that it was found to cause apoptosis in pancreatic cancer cells—it killed them. This is significant because a major challenge in pancreatic cancer treatment is the resistance of human pancreatic cancer cells to apoptosis.[64]

Soy was marketed in America after WWII when hostilities interrupted the flow of tropical oils from the South Pacific. We got sold a lot of *unfermented* soy, everything from soy oil and soy milk to blocks of tofu and soy baby formula. But meanwhile, the Japanese who had low rates of cancer, ate predominately *fermented* soy foods (natto,

63 Wainright W. The Management of Estrogens, Estrogen Receptors, Estrogen Metabolism, and Cellular Immunity in the Treatment of Cancers. *Townsend Letter*, Aug/Sept 2010, p.76-82

64 Rothe J, Wakileh M et al. The flavonoid beverage Haelan 951 induces growth arrest and apoptosis in pancreatic carcinoma cell lines in vitro. *BMC Complement Altern Med.* July 2015; 15: 212.

miso, tempeh). Every plant has enzyme inhibitors and anti-nutrient properties to protect it from predators and they cause problems for humans too. The soybean plant is especially rich in these chemicals. The traditional fermentation neutralizes these compounds and naturally adds protein, essential amino acids, essential fatty acids, vitamins, plus numerous antioxidants and phytosterols in the food.

I'll be honest: The taste of Haelan can be challenging. But here's the secret: Combine it with cinnamon, cacao powder, and chocolate-raspberry stevia drops. It makes a big difference.

- **GcMAF**

I have been curious about GcMAF because you hear great things about it, but it does not work for everyone. It is very distinct in its response and Dr. Rick Davis (www.QuickLab.com) explains it:

> In all of tumor biology, few molecules can claim to be more sublime, more effective, more controversial, or more important to human health than an obscure yet uniquely powerful activator of cellular immunity than the vitamin D-binding protein named GcMAF (a.k.a., Gc protein-derived Macrophage Activating Factor)."
>
> GcMAF is formed when three sugar molecules are sequentially cleaved away from the vitamin D / Gc precursor protein complex of surface receptors displayed on certain white blood cells called monocytes. GcMAF induces a Doctor Jekyll / Mr. Hyde transformation of these monocytes into an aggressive population of tumor and pathogen destroying cells called M2 macrophages ("big eaters"). M2 macrophages are the SEAL teams of our immune system. Their sole assignment is to seek out and destroy cancer cells, along with pathogenic viruses and bacteria. Every minute of every day M2 cells comb through every tissue in the body in recon missions looking for 'the bad guys.' When spotted, M2 cells attack their prey by engulfing them, then releasing powerful enzymes that literally digest them.
>
> Oh, if it were only that simple. Mother Nature can often be a cruel taskmaster. In the case of cancer, she has imbued them with an ability to defend themselves by releasing an enzyme of their own called nagalase which can intercept GcMAF-activated M2

THERAPY

cells and disable them by stripping away the GcMAF, thus converting the M2 cells back into harmless monocytes that simply pass by the invaders without taking notice.

So it is that our lives depend upon this lethal choreography of two dancers who are mortal enemies of each other. On the one hand, tumors secret nagalase as a means to evade immune system recognition, while on the other hand our bodies make GcMAF to recruit our M2 fighters to identify and kill cancer. It is a dynamic high-stakes battle of life and death—Le Danse Macabre—*The Dance of Death.*

- **Hydrazine sulfate**

Hydrazine Sulfate is a product developed by Dr. Joseph Gold of Syracuse University; clinical studies were begun in 1973.

Cancerous tumors produce lactic acid that is converted in the liver into glucose which the cancer cells then use as fuel. But that process takes a lot of energy and it explains the wasting syndrome that many cancer patients experience called cachexia—the cancer is thriving while the patient is literally starving to death. It is helpful to block the conversion process and hydrazine sulfate blocks a key enzyme in the liver that allows lactic acid to be converted into glucose. The use of hydrazine sulfate is a simple and very effective way to starve cancer. In the 1970s, Dr. Dean Burk of the National Cancer Institute called hydrazine sulfate "the most remarkable anticancer agent I have come across in my forty-five years of experience in cancer."[65] But the methods used by the "cancer establishment" to squash this all-too-effective therapy since then would make a great cloak-and-dagger novel.[66] You can order hydrazine sulfate here: http://www.positive-works.com/hydrazine.

- **Salicinium™**

Circulating tumor cells (CTCs) are at the forefront of a cancer that is spreading. Salicinium affects these cells first, thereby contributing

65 Pelton R. Overholser K. *Alternatives in Cancer Therapy: The Complete Guide to Alternative Treatments.* Simon & Schuster, 1994, p 139

66 Gold J. The Truth About Hydrazine Sulfate-Dr. Gold Speaks. July 2004. Accessed at www.hydrazinesulfate.org

THERAPY

to halting the spread of malignancy. Salicinium is a natural plant based extract, a complexed sugar molecule that is harmless to normal cells in the body because they cannot absorb a "complex glycome." Because this extract is a complexed molecule and not a "free" glucose, it has no impact on the patients' blood sugar. Cancer cells, however, falsely interpret the presence of this molecule as a sugar (a fuel source) and absorb it.

Cancer cells produce an enzyme called nagalase to cloak them from the immune system in order to avoid detection and destruction. Salicinium inhibits the production of nagalase while simultaneously stimulating the innate immune cells. The therapy can be delivered intravenously or orally but should be continued until the patient is cancer-clear.

Dr. Robert Eslinger (www.renointegrativemedicalcenter.com) is a leading integrative cancer physician who considers Salicinium a key component of his integrative program for cancer and chronic disease. He says, "I use Salicinium because it is a perfect marriage with IPT. When the sugar is low (therapeutic range), Salicinium (because it is a "fake sugar") is the perfect thing to present to the cancer just as it is getting desperate for sugar." He adds it to his IPT therapy, and uses it by itself on days when he does not use IPT. Inventor Joe Brown is now a researcher for Perfect Balance, the makers of Salicinium. Read more at http://www.salicinium.com.

- **Silver**

Many people with cancer have co-infections, especially of a viral and fungal nature. Silver is a time-honored tool for combating infections. It is a non-toxic, broad-spectrum antimicrobial therapy with no known toxicity and no known mechanism for acquired resistance. However, not all silver products are equal. We've all seen the result of poorly made products, those pictures of people whose skin turned gray—that's Argyria, a benign cosmetic condition caused when extreme amounts of silver are taken and the body tries to eliminate it by excreting it out through the skin. So small particle size and uniform

THERAPY

particle dispersion are critically important when choosing a high quality, effective silver product.

Here's a photo taken from a Transmission Electron Microscope of what good dispersion looks like—that's the one on the left and it shows the silver product Argentyn 23. The photo on the right, a different silver product sold through multi-level marketing channels, shows what bad dispersion (aggregation or clumping) looks like.

COMPARATIVE ANALYSIS

Sample I.D.	Claim PPM	Actual PPM	pH	Color	Conduct.
XX163B	18	20	7.48	Clear	23.1
Argentyn 23	23	23.13	6.69	Clear	19

Electron Microscopy

 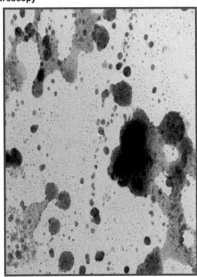

Argentyn 23   *<<< Micrographs are 100,000x magnification >>>*   **XX163B**

According to the company, "The huge solid masses of silver shown on the right illustrate how the vast majority of the silver is not on the surface, and thus chemically unavailable to participate as a bio-active species of silver. It is more beneficial to focus on the amount of bio-active silver present in a product rather than the size. The smaller the particle size, the more surface area there is to convert into bioactive silver, requiring positively-charged silver particles to release unbound silver ions. And again, it is the bio-active and bio-available form of silver that offers the practitioner a strategic immune-enhancing tool while being devoid of toxicity or side effects, as a result of the combination of the smallest unprecedented particle size of 0.8 nanometers and low concentration of 23 parts-per-million, as clearly demonstrated in the photograph to the left."

Argentyn 23 is my silver of choice. It is sold to professionals and many doctors in my foundation use it intravenously as well. The company sells a less potent version of Argentyn 23 to consumers; it is called Sovereign Silver and is found in health food stores.

- **Artemisinin/Artesunate**

Artemisinin is an herb used by the Chinese for thousands of years to treat malaria. In the 1970s, this herb and its semisynthetic derivative artesunate made their way into clinical use to treat drug resistant falciparum malaria and many cancers. When artemisinin/artesunate comes into contact with iron, it creates reactive free radicals that kill malaria parasites and cancer cells. Both cancer cells and malaria parasites sequester iron; they store up to 1000 times as much of it as what normal cells store. Giving artemisinin to people with malaria or cancer results in destruction of these abnormal cells and leaves normal cells unaffected.[67,68,69,70]

---

67 Efferth, Thomas et al. "Enhancement of cytotoxicity of artemisinins toward cancer cells by ferrous iron." *Free Radical Biology and Medicine* 37.7 (2004): 998-1009.

68 Du, Ji-Hui et al. "Artesunate induces oncosis-like cell death in vitro and has antitumor activity against pancreatic cancer xenografts in vivo." *Cancer chemotherapy and pharmacology* 65.5 (2010): 895-902.

69 MIYACHI, HAYATO, and CHRISTOPHER R. CHITAMBAR. "The anti-malarial artesunate is also active against cancer." *International journal of oncology* 18 (2001): 767-773.

70 Michaelis, Martin et al. "Anti-cancer effects of artesunate in a panel of chemoresistant neuroblastoma cell lines." *Biochemical pharmacology* 79.2 (2010): 130-136.

THERAPY

Bastyr Integrative Oncology Research Center recently found the high-dose IV Vitamin C in conjunction with IV artesunate makes a marked difference in advanced cancers. The artesunate is administered first, followed closely by the vitamin C. Conclusions have been drawn that artemisinin has chemo-like properties but it is also believed that high and frequent doses would be needed to actually replace chemotherapy.

I began using artemisinin capsules in 2003 upon the advice of my IPT physician. He told me that if I took it on an empty stomach, it could kill cancer with the effectiveness of chemotherapy but without the side-effects. My regimen: Upon awakening, first take my dose of ESSIAC tea, wait 5 minutes, and then take 2 capsules of artemisinin. I would wait 30 minutes before meals. At bedtime, at least 2 hours after meals, I did a second dose of artemisinin after ESSIAC tea.

- **Iscador/Mistletoe**

Mistletoe extract (Iscador) is used in Europe but not so much in the United States. It became better known after Suzanne Somers wrote that she uses it as an adjunctive therapy with breast cancer. It was Rudolf Steiner (1981-1925) who first said that mistletoe could be effective in the treatment of cancer. It is not seen as a cure but as a treatment used in conjunction with other conventional treatments. It is thought to slow the growth of tumors and prolong survival. I have not used it. Read more at http://www.steinerhealth.org/programs/cancer-treatment.

- **Laetrile**

The laetrile movement, founded in the 1950s by Ernst T. Krebs, Sr., was based on the idea that a chemical found naturally in the pits of apricots could fight tumors. Laetrile is a patented drug made from the natural compound amygdalin which is found in the seeds of many fruits and in almonds. Laetrile is also known as Amigdalina B-17 or vitamin B17. By 1978, it was estimated that more than 70,000 Americans had tried it—despite the fact it has been banned in the U.S. since 1963. There was a very controversial study done on laetrile in the 1970s at Sloan-Kettering (read about it at http://articles.mercola.com/

THERAPY

sites/articles/archive/2014/10/18/laetrile-cancer-research-cover-up. aspx). Subsequent studies showed it has potential to reduce the spread of cancer. Most people obtain laetrile from Tijuana clinics, as the agent is still legal in Mexico.

NOTE: I am as cautious these days about the prices at Mexican clinics as I am about U.S. clinics. Years ago, U.S. clinics charged more for services because they had higher overhead. In 2002 when I went to Mexico for treatment, the price was truly based on their overhead. It was a very affordable treatment compared to the U.S. Things have changed, however, and now it is a case of consumer beware. Most clinics in Mexico now want anywhere from $10,000 to $30,000 per week, and the programs tend to present themselves as "the solution." But cancer doesn't develop in three to six weeks, and it is not cured in three to six weeks.

- **3 Bromopyruvate (3BP)**

This is a lab-created molecule developed at John Hopkins University School of Medicine. It is an alkylating molecule that targets cancer cells' energy metabolism. But I want to put up a red flag here. Although it is an attractively fast acting cancer-killing agent, it also can be deadly. The molecule can be unstable. It is still in clinical trials; I for one do not want to be a guinea pig.

- **NuCalm®**

As referenced in the previous chapter, NuCalm is a machine, one proven to balance the autonomic nervous system. NuCalm acts like a reset button that calms and focuses your mind while allowing your body to recover. This system creates deep relaxation by mimicking patterns our brains recognize to help it relax. The technology works naturally with the two ways our brain communicates with our body—chemically and electrically. When we are in a deeply relaxed state, our bodies can heal and recover.

- **Budwig Protocol**

This cancer treatment is named for Dr. Johanna Budwig (1908-2003), a seven-time Nobel Prize nominee. She believed commercially

THERAPY

processed fats and oils—especially trans fats—destroy the natural electrical charge our cells use to work properly and then our cells start to suffocate due to a lack of oxygen. Chronic disease results. Cancer cells, for example, thrive in a no-oxygen environment. The Budwig protocol works to reverse this damage by restoring the natural electrical charge in cells, which in turn draws oxygen into the cells. Her protocol is based on freshly ground organic flax oil and organic low fat cottage cheese to reverse stagnated growth processes. Budwig felt that flax oil was the best, and that the protein in cottage cheese was necessary to help digest the fat. I don't agree that flax is best, but I do believe that restoration of good fats in the diet is crucial. For decades, the government and organizations like the American Heart Association have been pushing corn, soy, canola, and cottonseed oils that were never part of the human diet until the Industrial Revolution gave us the technology to mechanically refine and hydrogenate them. These manufactured oils gave us trans fats, and more recently interesterified fats, which poison our metabolism. Health begins at the cellular level. Our bodies are made up of cells with membranes that have a "lipid bilayer," meaning a fat wall to waterproof them. We absolutely need to give our bodies good fats to make those cells.

- **Cellect™**

This is a nutritional powder called Cellect that was developed by Fred Eichorn, N.D., president of the National Cancer Research Foundation. He studied what causes cellular mutations and cured himself of pancreatic cancer. According to Eichorn, "Cellect corrects the body's biochemistry and the environment to a level that is correct for normal cells, but is not conducive to cancer cells, and therefore the cancer cells die off as a result."

We know from soil testing that there are fewer minerals in the soil today than 100 years ago, so the plants we eat can't deliver as much nutrition. Add to that the amount of processed food in the diet and it is easy to see why nutrition tests indicate the average American is

THERAPY

woefully lacking in minerals and vitamins. The body needs these nutrients to do its many jobs properly. I don't use it, but it is very popular.

- **AvéULTRA®**

I first heard about AvéULTRA (aka Avemar® or Fermented Wheat Germ Extract or FWGE) from a cancer patient back in 2007; she was convinced it was improving her test results. According to the manufacturer, American BioSciences Inc., it has been the subject of more than 100 studies pertaining to in vitro (test tubes, petri dishes), in vivo (live animal or human tests) and human clinical trials. It has the following anti-cancer properties:

- Regulates glucose metabolism at the cellular level*
- Promotes immune system modulation*
- Maintains healthy cellular & humoral (Th1/Th2) immune balance*
- Promotes optimal NK cell targeting ability and the coordinated response of white blood cells: macrophages, B-cells, T-cells and NK cells*
- Enhances the ability of T-cells to respond to antigen presentation*
- Enhances the ability of B-cells to respond to activation and produce appropriate antibodies*

* These statements have not been approved by the FDA.

Fermented Wheat Germ Extract (FWGE) is available as a freeze-dried powder that comes in pre-measured packets. When I hear about FWGE from patients, it is usually to say that they cannot tolerate the taste. The company has remedied this by developing Fermented Wheat Germ Extract—Super Concentrate that comes in a pill form under the name Metatrol® (and Metatrol Pro® for professionals). According to the company, Metatrol and Metatrol Pro are the most potent and super-concentrated forms of FWGE available. The daily dose is two capsules you can easily swallow. None of the fermented wheat germ extract products contain gluten.

THERAPY

- **ESSIAC® Tea**

This beverage is a combination of three blood purifying herbs and one anti-cancer herb. I first learned about ESSIAC tea in 1993 when I was sick with the Myalgic Encephalomyelitis. ESSIAC tea was developed by a Canadian nurse name Renee Caisse; ESSIAC is her name spelled backwards. Nurse Caisse got the basics of the formula from the Ojibway Indians whom she noticed had low evidence of cancer and disease. The Indians used eight herbs (burdock, sheep sorrel, slippery elm, turkey rhubarb, red clover, watercress, goldthread, and periwinkle), but Nurse Caisse refined the formula to just four.

The four organic herbs are burdock root, Turkish rhubarb root, slippery elm, and sheep sorrel. They are steeped into water to make a tea. The sheep sorrel is the anti-cancer herb. In my experience, the commercially prepared versions of ESSIAC tea are not that effective; some versions do not even have the right ingredients. I learned recently, to my chagrin, that not only was the bottled tincture I had been using not effective enough, but I should have been making the tea with the sheep sorrel herb along with its roots. According to Rene Caisse, leaving out the sheep sorrel root is leaving out the most important ingredient. I found a great site for the herbs, and the sheep sorrel includes the roots. They have everything necessary to make ESSIAC, including equipment to brew the tea: http://renecaissetea.com.

- **Red Clover Stillingia (AKA The Hoxsey Formula)**

Red clover is a plant that grows wild in Europe and has been naturalized to grow in the United States. The University of Maryland Medical Center states, "Based on its traditional use for cancer, researchers have begun to study the role of isoflavones from red clover in cancer prevention and treatment. Preliminary evidence suggests these isoflavones may stop cancer cells from growing or kill cancer cells in test tubes. Researchers theorize that red clover may help prevent some forms of cancer, such as prostate and endometrial cancer. However, because of the herb's estrogen-like effects, it might also contribute to the growth of some cancers, just as estrogen does. Until further research is done, doctors cannot recommend red clover to prevent cancer. Women with a history of breast cancer should not take red clover."[71]

This raises a valid concern, just like unfermented soy and flax, regarding the wisdom of introducing even more estrogens in the body in an era when we are flooded with so many environmental estrogens—synthetic substances that when absorbed into the body, function similarly to estrogen (plastics, pesticides, detergents, preservatives, etc.)

That said, red clover is only part of the Hoxsey Formula. The Hoxsey Formula was brought to the world of cancer by Harry Hoxsey, the son of a veterinarian who used the therapy on horses in the early 1920s. Although he saw many people completely turn their cancer around, the medical establishment hounded him persistently. According to Ty Bollinger, creator of the The Truth About Cancer series:

> Hoxsey's treatments were considered effective by a panel of independent physicians who had reviewed the case histories of his patients. Their written testimonies were used in Hoxsey's 1950 lawsuit against the AMA, along with testimonials from some of his cured patients. His tonics were meant to help create homeostasis (internal stability), kill cancer cells, and remove the toxins created from killing cancer cells. This perspective is in line with almost all natural cancer treatments and practitioners today.

The therapy consists of two formulas. The external salve is a red paste made with bloodroot (an anti-tumor ingredient) mixed with zinc chloride and antimony sulfide that is applied directly onto skin cancer tumors. Then there is an internal tonic consisting of red clover blossom, licorice root, buckthorn bark, burdock root, stillingia root, poke root, barberry root, Oregon grape root, cascara sagrada bark, prickly ash bark, wild Indigo root, and sea kelp. The sea kelp may have been added more recently to the original formula. A supplement of potassium iodide was included along with the tonic.

---

71 University of Maryland Medical Center. Accessed at http://umm.edu/health/medical/altmed/herb/red-clover

There has been no definitive study of the Hoxsey formula, but there are several studies that indicate that some of its ingredients may have antitumor effects. The Hoxsey Therapy can still be received at the Bio-Medical Center in Tijuana, Mexico.

- **Pau d'arco**

Pau d'arco is a South American herb that has been used to treat a variety of conditions including candida, arthritis, pain, inflammation of the prostate gland, ulcers, dysentery, fevers, and cancer. The University of Maryland Medical School states that there were reported medical uses of pau d'arco as early as 1873.[72] Pau d'arco is a potent anti-microbial, and must be used with due respect. Most of the studies in pau d'arco are centered on the heartwood of the tree. However most of the commercially available products contain the inner and the outer bark of the tree. This may explain varying results in people who use it. You can read more at http://www.herb-care.com.

I included pau d'arco in my program early on. At the time, I bought a bag of the herb in powder form and made my own tea. It was not a good-tasting tea, but I drank it faithfully. Since then, I have learned that you must make sure that the inner bark of the tree (the most potent part) has been used in the preparation of the supplement, tea, or lotion. Tea is the original form and here's a good site for how to make it, and they confirm that they use the inner bark. http://store.renecaissetea.com/collections/essiac-tea-herbs/products/pau-d-arco-8-oz

- **Modified Citrus Pectin**

This is a supplement from ecoNugenics® with multiple benefits. The pectin is derived from the pith of lemons, limes, oranges, and grapefruit. No juice, pulp or any other part of the fruit is used.

Modified citrus pectin (MCP) is a specialized fruit polysaccharide. It has shown unique properties in blocking cancer cell aggregation, adhesion, and metastasis[73] because of its effect on a galactin-3. That

---

72 http://umm.edu/health/medical/altmed/herb/pau-darco

73 Modified citrus pectin-monograph. Altern Med Rev. 2000 Dec;5(6):573-5. Accessed at http://www.ncbi.nlm.nih.gov/pubmed/11134980

is a molecule, a rogue protein, normally present in the body at low concentrations. However, when elevated in circulation, galactin-3 is recognized as a chief culprit in the advancement of life-threatening illnesses involving inflammation and fibrosis, as well as metastatic cancer.

According to Dr. Dr Isaac Eliaz who formulates PectaSol-C®, the brand of MCP used in studies and clinical trials, galectin-3 is over-expressed on the surface of cancer cells, acting as a sticky surface molecule which allows cancer cells to aggregate, disseminate throughout the circulatory system, evade immune surveillance, and establish themselves at distant sites. It is also involved in angiogenesis. "Controlling excess galectin-3," he said, "can result in significant benefits and help prevent the advancement of cancer and other life-threatening diseases. MCP is a proven galectin-3 antagonist, a natural inhibitor of this molecule, and thus it helps control cancer development and metastasis, and reduces inflammation and fibrosis."

It is shown to help limit disease progression in men with advanced prostate cancer.[74] In terms of longevity, MCP is poised to significantly reduce the odds of a secondary or metastatic cancers. Life Extension Magazine reports:[75]

> As scientists begin to decipher the process of how cells receive, interpret, and relay the signals that recruit them to form new tumors,[76] they are focusing their attention on molecules called galactose-binding lectins, or *galectins*. Galectins are overexpressed adhesion and blood vessel-attracting surface molecules that are thought to be involved in the spread of cancer...[77]

---

74 Azemar M, Hildenbrand B, et al. Clinical benefit in patients with advanced solid tumors with modified citrus pectin: a prospective pilot study. *Clin Med: Oncol.* 2007;1:73–80.

75 Nicholas J. Fighting Cancer Metastasis and Heavy Metal Toxicities With Modified Citrus Pectin. *Life Extension Magazine*, March 2009

76 Gupta GP, Massague J. Cancer metastasis: building a framework. Cell. 2006 Nov 17;127(4):679-95.

77 Glinskii OV, Huxley VH, Glinsky GV, et al. Mechanical entrapment is insufficient and intercellular adhesion is essential for metastatic cell arrest in distant organs. *Neoplasia.* 2005 May;7(5):522-7.

THERAPY

Via the mechanism of *galectin-3 antagonism,* MCP appears to disrupt the processes that allow cancer cells to communicate with one another. When the MCP molecules bind to receptors on the surface of cancer cells, they block galectin-3 and other molecules from penetrating into nearby healthy tissue to create a new tumor and establish the tumor's blood supply (angiogenesis). In this way, MCP seems to play a role in preventing cancerous tumors from metastasizing and spreading to other organs—one of the main causes of death from cancer.

Research shows that modified citrus pectin also can have an effect in chelating toxic heavy metals, which I believe add to the toxic overload that contributes to cancer. And it chelates without affecting mineral levels.

PectaSol-C® MCP comes both in capsules and as a powder. You take it on an empty stomach. They make a lime flavored powder and I think it tastes so good, it's almost like drinking a lemonade in the middle of the day—minus the sugar, of course. (They use stevia.)

- **Mushroom Extracts**

Medicinal mushrooms are powerful remedies that can help bring back one's pep, vitality, and enthusiasm for life. So how is a fungus like the mushroom an anti-cancer medicine for a disease that likes a fungal state? Dr. Nalini Chilkov (www.nalinichilkov.com) explains:

Just as there are bacteria that cause disease and infection, there are bacteria, such as the friendly bacteria living in our intestines that actually help us to fight disease, manage inflammation, detoxify our hormones and more. In exactly the same way there are fungi that are pathogenic and contribute to fungal infection, illness and disease, and there are also fungi that are medicinal and therapeutic and healing and fight disease. These therapeutic, medicinal and healing mushrooms include but are not limited to Cordyceps (Turkey Tail), Coriolus, Ganoderma (Reishi) , Poria, Agaricus, and more. Even the common button mushrooms we eat in our salads contain powerful beta gluons, polysaccharides and fatty acids that have positive, not negative effects upon our health. In Asia the more tasty medicinal mushrooms are also included in many dishes. For example, you will find the delicious Shiitake mushrooms available fresh or dried. Including these mushrooms makes your food medicine.

Dr. Martha Grout (www.arizonaadvancedmedicine.com) points out that most forests depend upon the presence, abundance, and variety of mushrooms and their interconnecting roots. Mushrooms produce a network of roots called the "mycelium" which is packed with vitamins and nutrients, helps to condition the soil in which it grows, helps choose beneficial bacteria to break down nutrients, and helps produce other nutrients which we human beings cannot produce ourselves:

> Mushrooms and their mycelia have been shown to be prebiotics for our gut, encouraging the growth of helpful bacteria like Acidophilus and Bifidobacterium, as well as supporting our immune systems. For medicinal purposes, mushrooms have been shown to activate Toll-like receptors, a very important part of the innate immune system which is also involved in recognition of cancerous cells, and preventing their growth.[78] Get your mushrooms—both food and medicinal—grown organically, so that you may get the benefit of their ability to clean up *your* toxic environment.

At the 2011 Annie Appleseed Conference, Mark Kaylor stated that three different mushrooms have a dramatic effect for better health:

1. Eating 9 to 12 shitake mushrooms a day is an anti-fungal that also revitalizes the liver.

2. Chaga mushrooms are extraordinarily strong and show great promise for strengthening your constitution. In fact, the body of the 5,000-year-old "Iceman" of the Alps was found with a medicine pouch containing similar mushrooms.

3. Kaylor's favorite is the reishi mushroom, which is good for sleep, and for the heart, lungs, liver, kidneys—just about everything.

THERAPY

78 Kasai H, He LM et al. IL-12 Production Induced by Agaricus blazei Fraction H (ABH) Involves Toll-like Receptor (TLR). *Evid Based Complement Alternat Med.* 2004 Dec;1(3):259-267.

Dr. Chilkov's favorite mushroom for cancer patients is the Cordyceps sinensis (CS), a tradition in Chinese Medicine and a fungus that has been used for over 2000 years as part of a treatment for a variety of conditions including many cancers. She suggests that Cordyceps is best taken as either a tea or soup; also a high quality powder can be mixed into juice or water, yogurt, or applesauce.

Available evidence suggests that the efficacy of CS as a potential anti-neoplastic/anti-cancer therapeutic agent is related to a role as an activator of innate immune responses. Studies show the following actions and effects of the water extract of CS:[79]

- The polysaccharides in CS have been shown to have immune stimulating and anti-tumor activity.

- CS had been shown to inhibit the growth of several cancer cell lines.

- CS has also been shown to protect the liver and kidneys from toxic side effects of chemotherapy.

- CS has been shown to potentiate and enhance the activity of some chemotherapy drugs.

- CS has been shown to promote cell death (induce apoptosis). Normal cells will self-destruct (undergo apoptosis) when the cell is damaged. Cancer cells fail to do so. Agents which cause normal cell death are used widely in chemotherapy today. CS has been shown to induce apoptosis or normal cell death in cancer cells in many studies and suggests that CS might be a valuable adjunct therapy for cancer patients.

- CS is a potent antioxidant, thus protecting cells from free radical damage. Free radical damage is a process in which free electrons damage our cells and our DNA and is thought to be a primary factor in the aging process. Additionally when DNA (genetic material)

THERAPY

---

79 http://www.integrativecanceranswers.com/cordyceps-cancer-support-and-immune-modulation-from-an-ancient-chinese-herbal-medicine/

in the cells is damaged, risk of cancer increases. CS has been shown to enhance the production of Glutathione and SOD, protective, natural antioxidants produced in our cells to protect against free radical damage and oxidation.

- CS demonstrates anti-inflammatory properties. Inflammation is a factor common to many diseases, including cancer. Supporting the management of inflammation modulates our immune system. In particular, CS has been shown to suppress the production of COX-2, NFkB and TNFa, inflammatory molecules present in cancer cells and many other disease processes.

- CS has been shown to increase the production of Natural Killer (NK) cells. NK cells are primary protective cell in our natural innate immune response is active against both tumor cells and viral cells.

- CS has also been shown to inhibit metastasis and the spread of some cancers. It is metastasis, the spread of cancer cells from the primary original site of the tumor to other parts of the body that causes cancer patients to die. Inhibiting metastasis therefore prolong life for cancer patients.

- Some studies have shown that CS prevents metastasis by inhibiting angiogenesis, the process by which tumor cells make new blood vessels, allowing tumors to grow in size as well as allowing cancer cells to enter the blood stream and travel to other parts of the body.

- Qualitatively cancer patients using CS along with their chemotherapy report less fatigue, reduced pain and less weight loss during treatment.

- CS has also demonstrated anti-viral and antibacterial properties. Cancer patients are often at risk for infection during chemotherapy and after surgery. Researchers hypothesize that CS increases resistance to infections by modulating immune function, increasing white blood cells and Natural Killer cells and by modulating inflammation.

THERAPY

- Additionally, CS has been shown to protect against bone loss and osteoporosis, a risk factor for many patients, especially breast cancer and prostate cancer patients on medications that block hormones.

- **KAQUN Water**

KAQUN Water (pronounced ca-<u>coon</u>) is the result of 20 years of research and is the only known water to have undergone 10+ years of clinical and laboratory research carried out on both healthy volunteers and those with health challenges, as well as animal studies. With KAQUN technology, no chemicals or toxic materials are used; using water as the source, oxygen is made into a stabilized form with concentrations of 18-25 mg per liter.

There are two forms of KAQUN water delivered to the body: the KAQUN baths or the milder KAQUN drinking water. I went to Hungary in 2014 to investigate this water. The baths were like nothing I have ever experienced before. The water was so oxygenated it was extremely buoyant; it is purported to have taken an O_2 molecule and enhanced it to an O_{126} strength. The water was so buoyant I could not get my body down to the bottom of the tub for a large part of the 50-minute session. When I finished with the bath, my skin was plump and hydrated and smooth. I am a diabetic, and so when I have sores they last for a long time. The sores—which usually would take weeks to heal—were healed within four baths. I felt energized and ready to take on most anything the day had to offer, and at night I slept really well.

The drinking water (O_{64} strength) also filled me with oxygen, and I had responses to it that you would imagine one would have from high oxygen and alkalinity, including some detoxification.

While I was in Hungary, I had a chance to look at some of their clinical response pictures. I saw radiation and other burn victims' before and after pictures, and they were pretty amazing. But they also had case studies of cancer patients who experienced great remissions. It was very encouraging.

There are many KAQUN baths in Hungary. Currently, there are no baths in the United States or anywhere else in the world, although there are many distributors of the drinking water and gel internationally. This is not water that has been alkalinized or given an electrical charge. This is about a transformed molecule with a highly-bound oxygen content. To learn more about KAQUN or to find a distributor, visit www.kaqun.eu.

- **Selenium Therapy**

Selenium is a trace mineral that used to be pretty available in our diet because it used to be plentiful in the soil. But modern farming techniques tend to sterilize the soil and we don't get the amount of selenium we used to. One of the best food sources is the Brazil nut.

This mineral works in conjunction with vitamin E, vitamin C, glutathione, and vitamin B3 as an antioxidant to prevent free radical damage in the body. It's thought to help prevent cancer by affecting oxidative stress, inflammation, and DNA repair.

Selenium was first noted as a cancer treatment in medical journals more than 100 years ago. Nutritional historian Chris Barr—who considers selenium "the best answer for cancer"—has been studying the effects of selenium on cancer. According to Barr, 900 micrograms and up to 2,000 mcg a day will achieve normal blood selenium levels in terminal cancer patients and can bring about remissions.

> The form of selenium used was the whole food, grown variety. It was given to 141 patients among which eight had lung cancer and were given only six months to live. At the end of one year, four of those terminal lung cancer patients were still alive. At the end of four years there were 103 terminal cancer patients still alive who were all supposed to have died within the first year.

- **DMSO**

Dimethyl Sulfoxide (DMSO) has been a by-product of the wood industry and has been in use as a commercial solvent since 1953. Even though in 125 countries throughout the world, including Canada, Great Britain, Germany, and Japan, doctors prescribe it for a variety of ailments, including pain, inflammation, scleroderma, interstitial

THERAPY

cystitis, and arthritis elevated intracranial pressure, and some 11,000 articles have been written on its medical and clinical implications, the FDA has approved it only for use as a preservative of organs for transplant and for interstitial cystitis, a disease of the bladder.

The National Cancer Institute reports the results of a 1996 study in which treatment with DMSO causes a significant prolongation of the host's life-time expectancy.[80] Although it has been 20 years since that study, and all the studies listed above have been performed, DMSO is still not approved for use for cancer and chronic disease. So we turn again to off-label use.

I have used DMSO as a spray and an ointment, as well as receiving it via IV. There was a doctor many years ago who used DMSO with fractionated doses of chemotherapy as a modified IPT. He called it DPT, or DMSO Potentiated Therapy. DMSO can bind to Adriamycin, vinblastine, 5-fluorouracil (i.e. 5-Fu), and cisplatin per the Oregon Health Sciences University.

Dr. Jonathan Murphy (www.anoasisofhealing.com) explains it like this: "DMSO is two methyl groups (-CH3) attached like Mickey Mouse ears on the side of a sulfur-oxygen molecule. It is very simple and is carried mostly everywhere in the body, so it goes right through the skin the cell walls, and the blood brain barrier. It is also an excellent solvent, so it can dissolve and deliver other things throughout the body. In its own right, it is a strong antioxidant which can neutralize free radicals." And to prevent metastases? "Nests of cancer cells flake off of tumors and are known as circulating tumor cells when flowing in the bloodstream. These are not so easily implanted into otherwise healthy tissue when DMSO, a strong antioxidant, is dissolved in the blood and other body tissue fluids. DMSO is an excellent solvent which crosses all membranes so its own right DMSO can reach any cells in the body and so can have their effect on metastases everywhere. Although it is

80 Bergamo A, Cocchietto M, Capozzi I, Mestroni G, Alessio E, Sava G. Treatment of Residual Metastases with Na[trans-RuC14 (DMSO)lm] and Ruthenium Uptake by Tumor Cells. *PubMed* 1996 Aug;7(6):697-702.

frowned on by the FDA, DMSO can potentiate other agents including chemotherapy agents."

- **Functional Integrative Dentistry**

Note that I did not title this section "Biological Dentistry." There is a paradigm shift happening where it is becoming more widely understood that what happens in the mouth, does not stay in the mouth. When teeth are pulled, improperly healed holes in the jawbone called cavitations occur upwards of 80 percent of the time. Think of a cavitation as a little cesspool, constantly dripping bits of infectious material into the body which distract the immune system from bigger jobs, say, identifying and killer cancer cells. As the medical community better accepts the idea that the mouth is part of the rest of the body, functional dentistry is taking its rightful place within the larger picture of functional medicine. As Mathew Steinberg, D.D.S. (www.drmatthewsteinberg.com) puts it:

> We are now becoming the physicians of the oral cavity. Dentists do not just look for cavities anymore, but now examine, screen, and help to co-diagnose breathing and airway disorders, as well as periodontal gum and bone disease which can have a direct influence on every organ in the body because toxic bacteria can invade organs such as the heart, lungs and pancreas and set up sites for disease. Dentists can now use new fluorescent light technology to screen for oral cancer. A disease free oral environment, and that includes the mouth, is so important to a healthy quality of life that it can add up to an additional 10 years to one's lifespan.

Dr. Hal Huggins, an early leader in this paradigm shift, described the average practice of dentistry as toxic—mercury fillings, fluoride rinses, and root canals performed with no respect for their impact on the body's meridians. As he explained at our BAFC annual conference in 2012:

> Elsewhere in medicine, when a body part dies, it is cut out or amputated. In dentistry, however, a dead tooth is left in the

THERAPY

mouth. We have necrotic (dead) tissue in root canals and dentin tubules, and we have no way to get into these canals and clean this tissue out. Strep, staph, and 92 other bacteria love necrotic tissue. You can kill the bacteria with ozone or Sanum remedies but you cannot remove the dead corpses—their DNA is still there. It's like in war—you can kill the soldier but his gun is not dead; someone else can pick it up and use that. A harmless bacterium can 'swallow' that DNA and become a pathogen.

Cancer patients, who have an incompetent immune system, really benefit from working with a dentist who understands these kinds of holistic concepts.

- **Mind-body Medicine**

We have already explored the power of the mind over the body in Chapter XI, but I believe it bears repeating. In my opinion, this is a very underestimated, overlooked and, in most cases, unrecognized tool. In our anxiousness to grab and embrace the medical treatments that would rid our bodies of cancer, we overlook this one that is right at hand and totally FREE.

Brenda Stockdale, Director of Behavioral Medicine, Vantage Oncology/RCOG, has spent years helping integrate mind-body medicine into cancer clinics. She said, "Recent advances in science reveal we can learn to harness the healing power of the human spirit to positively influence most any condition. For cancer care to be truly comprehensive it requires that we implement this new understanding—both as patients and as practitioners—becoming responsible participants in our own healing process and in our lives." You can read up on this in her book, *You Can Beat the Odds: Surprising Factors Behind Chronic Illness & Cancer*.

Remember that the body listens to thoughts and beliefs. When I was diagnosed, I had no signs or symptoms of cancer. I felt perfectly fine. Because the situation was so unbelievable to me, I had the thought that the hospital had mixed up my biopsy with someone else's, and that some poor woman was walking around thinking she was fine when in

THERAPY

fact she had cancer. When the doctor said the scans showed lesions in my brain and lungs, I dismissed those findings; the lung lesions could be from my many bouts with bronchitis, and the brain lesions could have been caused by the ME.

But it was even more than that. On that first night, the night of the biopsy when I heard God, I arrived at the conclusion that no matter what—whether I lived or died—I was going to be okay. From that point on, that was my foundation. I had no real fundamental worries.

I'm convinced that one of the main reasons I am alive is my belief systems and my refusal to accept what the doctors said.

• Amino Acid Supplementation

Amino acids are the building blocks of proteins, and proteins are the building blocks of many tissues in the body. Proteins are also enzymes, hormones, and antibodies. We don't want to be short of any of those things.

Dr. David Minkoff stressed the importance of amino acids for cancer at the BAFC annual conference:

> Almost all cancer patients are low in essential amino acids and don't know it and neither do their doctors. But if you measure serum essential amino acids, some or all will be very low. In this state there will be diminished immune function as well as slowed detoxification and leaky membranes that make the patient susceptible to infection and toxin entry into the core of the body. When patients are replenished with the correct blend of essential amino acids they gain significant lean body mass and improve survival.

It makes sense to me to gain lean body mass, and it's a wonderful bonus that it has been known to improve survival. As with all supplements, I will get guidance from a health practitioner, most likely Dr. Minkoff in this case.

• Seeds

Yes, I said seeds, another concept that was introduced at the BAFC annual conferences. Dr. Bradford Weeks explained that "the seed is the

THERAPY

most nutrient dense food on earth—30x more nutrients in the seed compared to the rest of the fruit. Eating the (organic, non-GMO) seed is like feasting in the most exclusive VIP section of Mother Nature's restaurant. Nourish the body well and, in turn, the body performs miracles and restores its health better than any doctor."

Particular attention should be paid to the "black seed" also known as black cumin, black sesame, black caraway, onion seed, or Roman coriander. The earliest record of its cultivation and use come from ancient Egypt and was in fact found in Egyptian pharaoh Tutankhamen's tomb dating back 3,300 years ago.[81] There is a belief that that the Islamic prophet Mohammed said of it that it is "a remedy for all diseases except death."

Black cumin seed (botanical name Nigella sativa) has 16 documented benefits:

1. Prevents radiation damage: Nigella sativa oil (NSO) and its active component, thymoquinone, protect brain tissue from radiation-induced nitrosative stress.[82]

2. Protects against damage from heart attack[83]

3. Prevents morphine dependence/toxicity[84]

---

81 *Domestication of Plants in the Old World* (3 ed.). Oxford University Press. 2000. p. 206. ISBN 0-19-850356-3.

82 Adem Ahlatci, Abdurahman Kuzhan, Seyithan Taysi, Omer Can Demirtas, Hilal Eryigit Alkis, Mehmet Tarakcioglu, Ali Demirci, Derya Caglayan, Edibe Saricicek, Kadir Cinar. Radiation-modifying abilities of Nigella sativa and Thymoquinone on radiation-induced nitrosative stress in the brain tissue. *Phytomedicine*. 2013 Nov 21. pii: S0944-7113(13)00432-7. doi: 10.1016/j. phymed.2013.10.023.

83 Randhawa MA, Alghamdi MS et al. The effect of thymoquinone, an active component of Nigella sativa, on isoproterenol induced myocardial injury. *Pak J Pharm Sci*. 2013 Nov;26(6):1215-9.

84 Anvari M, Seddigh A et al. Nigella sativa extract affects conditioned place preference induced by morphine in rats. *Anc Sci Life*. 2012 Oct-Dec; 32(2): 82–88 doi: 10.4103/0257-7941.118537

4. Prevents kidney damage associated with diabetes: A thymoquinone extract from nigella sativa has protective effects on experimental diabetic nephropathy.[85]

5. Prevents post-surgical adhesions[86]

6. Prevents Alzheimer's associated neurotoxicity[87]

7. Suppresses breast cancer growth: A thymoquinone extract from nigella sativa inhibits tumor growth and induces programmed cell death (apoptosis) in a breast cancer xenograft mouse model.[88,89]

8. Exhibits anti-psoriasis properties[90]

9. Prevents brain pathology associated with Parkinson's disease[91]

85 Omran, OM. Effects of Thymoquinone on STZ-induced Diabetic Nephropathy: An Immunohistochemical Study. *Ultrastruct Pathol.* 2013 Oct 17.

86 Sahbaz A et al. Effect of Nigella sativa oil on postoperative peritoneal adhesion formation. *J Obstet Gynaecol Res.* 2013 Oct 7. doi: 10.1111/jog.12172.

87 Ismail N, Ismail M et al. Thymoquinone Preventsβ-Amyloid Neurotoxicity in Primary Cultured Cerebellar Granule Neurons. *Cell Mol Neurobiol.* 2013 Nov;33(8):1159-69. doi: 10.1007/s10571-013-9982-z. Epub 2013 Oct 8.

88 Woo CC, Annie Hsu, Alan Prem Kumar, Gautam Sethi, Kwong Huat Benny Tan. Thymoquinone Inhibits Tumor Growth and Induces Apoptosis in a Breast Cancer Xenograft Mouse Model: The Role of p38 MAPK and ROS. *PLoS One.* 2013 Oct 2;8(10):e75356. doi: 10.1371/journal.pone.0075356. PMID

89 Rajput S et al. Molecular targeting of Akt by thymoquinone promotes G1 arrest through translation inhibition of cyclin D1 and induces apoptosis in breast cancer cells. *Life Sci.* 2013 Nov 13;93(21):783-90. doi: 10.1016/j.lfs.2013.09.009. Epub 2013 Sep 15. PMID: 24044882

90 Dwarampudi L et al. Antipsoriatic activity and cytotoxicity of ethanolic extract of Nigella sativa seeds. *Pharmacogn Mag.* 2012 Oct-Dec; 8(32): 268–272. doi: 10.4103/0973-1296.103650

91 Alhebshi AH et al. Thymoquinone protects cultured hippocampal and human induced pluripotent stem cells-derived neurons againstα-synuclein-induced synapse damage. *Neurosci Lett.* 2013 Sep 27. pii: S0304-3940(13)00873-2. doi: 10.1016/j.neulet.2013.09.049.

THERAPY

10. Kills highly aggressive gliobastoma brain cancer cells: A thymo-quinone extract from nigella sativa exhibits glioblastoma cell killing activity.[92]

11. Kills leukemia cells: A thymoquinone from nigella sativa induces mitochondria-mediated apoptosis in acute lympho-blastic leukaemia in vitro.[93]

12. Suppresses liver cancer growth: A thymoquinone extract from nigella sativa prevents chemically-induced cancer in a rat model.[94]

13. Prevents diabetic pathologies: A water and alcohol extract of nigella sativa at low doses has a blood-sugar lowering effect and ameliorative effect on regeneration of pancreatic islets, indicating its value as a therapeutic agent in the management of diabetes mellitus.[95]

14. Suppresses cervical cancer cell growth: A thymoquinone extract from nigella sativa exhibits anti-proliferative, apoptotic and anti-invasive properties in a cervical cancer cell line.[96]

---

92 Racoma IO, Meisen WH et al. Thymoquinone inhibits autophagy and induces cathepsin-mediated, caspase-independent cell death in glioblastoma cells. *PLoS One*. 2013 Sep 9;8(9):e72882. doi: 10.1371/journal.pone.0072882.

93 Salim LZA, Mohan S et al. Thymoquinone induces mitochondria-mediated apoptosis in acute lymphoblastic leukaemia in vitro. *Molecules*. 2013 Sep 12;18(9):11219-40. doi: 10.3390/molecules180911219. PMID

94 Raghunandhakumar S, Paramasivam A et al. Selvam Senthilraja, Chandrasekar Naveenkumar, Selvamani Asokkumar, John Binuclara, Sundaram Jagan, Thymoquinone inhibits cell proliferation through regulation of G1/S phase cell cycle transition in N-nitrosodiethylamine-induced experimental rat hepatocellular carcinoma. *Toxicol Lett*. 2013 Oct 23;223(1):60-72. doi: 10.1016/j.toxlet.2013.08.018. Epub 2013 Sep 3. PMID

95 Alimohammadi S, Hobbenaghi R et al. Protective and antidiabetic effects of extract from Nigella sativa on blood glucose concentrations against streptozotocin (STZ)-induced diabetic in rats: an experimental study with histopathological evaluation. *Diagnostic Pathology*. 2013 8:137

96 Sakalar C, Yuruk M et al. Pronounced transcriptional regulation of apoptotic and TNF-NF-kappa-B signaling genes during the course of thymoquinone mediated apoptosis in HeLa cells. *Mol Cell Biochem*. 2013 Nov;383(1-2):243-51. doi: 10.1007/s11010-013-1772-x. Epub 2013 Aug 14.

THERAPY

15. Prevents lead-induced brain damage.[97]

16. Kills oral cancer cells: A thymoquinone extract from nigella sativa induces programmed cell death (apoptosis) in oral cancer cells.[98]

I've heard black cumin seed can taste gross. I get mine in a liquid form because I take so many pills I don't want to have to add another pill to the regime. It is called SOUL and it is a network marketing product. This is one example of when I am willing to pay for convenience. They also make a green drink called CORE which is a convenient, tasty way to get a dose of green drink every day. You can purchase SOUL and CORE at http://www.myrainlife.com/bestanswer.

• **Food**

Often when people think of cancer therapies, they think of drugs. But food is also a targeted cancer therapy—and a powerful one. Learn to add medicinal spices and herbs—turmeric is a great one—with every meal. Mushrooms, spicy peppers, onions, garlic, mustard, Brazil nuts, cruciferous vegetables are all anti-cancer. And tasty too!!!

Some of these targeted therapies can be used at home; some require a clinical setting and if you want to find an integrative physician, go here: http://bestanswerforcancer.org. Just under the butterfly logo, click on the button for "Find a Physician."

Many of the physicians named in this chapter are members of the International Organization of Integrative Cancer Physicians (IOICP). The Best Answer for Cancer Foundation certifies IOICP physicians in integrative oncology practices.

---

97 Radad K, Hassanein K et al. Thymoquinone ameliorates lead-induced brain damage in Sprague Dawley rats. PMID: 23910425

98 Abdelfadil E, Cheng YH et al. Thymoquinone induces apoptosis in oral cancer cells through p38β inhibition.

THERAPY

This targeted therapy modality is where you will need to be especially careful to chart your start and stop dates, and have staggered intervals. Remember that cancer is very intelligent about things that are trying to kill it. In fact, the only way in which I can see that cancer is stupid is that it eventually kills its host—us. So don't do any one thing for long enough for cancer to build immunity against it.

In the following NOTES section, write down your plan for your Timing Chart of duration/switching of foods and supplements. Are you going to take these notes directly to a physical calendar, and online calendar, or a calendar app? How are you going to be reminded that it is time to switch a supplement, food, or practice?

_____

_____

_____

_____

_____

_____

_____

Now start investigating targeted cancer therapies. Look for evidence-based medicine or for years of anecdotal histories behind each therapy. If you find a therapy that you like, look for a clinic that offers that therapy. Arrange to send in your medical records for a consultation; you will want to know if they have a plan specifically for you. If possible, you will want to talk to previous patients. Remember that if it is a new, unproven therapy, you are merely a sort of human guinea pig.

Best Answer for Cancer Foundation (BAFC) has a physician division called the International Organization of Integrative Cancer Physicians (IOICP), and offers an online directory of physicians who provide integrative and functional support for patients of cancer and chronic disease. When I was diagnosed in 2001, it was almost impossible to find qualified integrative physicians that had any kind of organization behind them for support and education. This organization and database exist specifically for that reason.

You can search the directory by going to www.bestanswerforcancer.org and clicking on "Find a Physician." The directory offers a search capability that lets you either look at all the integrative physician members or zero in to the physicians that are trained and certified in the targeted low-dose therapy, IPT/IPTLD. The physicians in the directory have all been vetted for education, licensure, and efforts in Continuing Medical Education.

THERAPY

_____

_____

_____

_____

_____

_____

_____

_____

_____

_____

_____

_____

_____

THERAPY

_____

_____

CHAPTER XVII

How Can You Make a Difference?

*W*hether you are a cancer patient, survivor, caregiver, or just an interested party reading this book, there are things you can do to help others, give back, and make a difference. Here are just a few suggestions:

Spread the word

Tell people about this book. Share information you have learned, and send them our website link www.bestanswerforcancer.org. Tell people they can find integrative physicians on our website who practice patient-centered medicine—putting the patient first and addressing the whole person.

Join our Group

Get on our mailing list by going to this link on your computer www.bestanswerforcancer.org/join. We will keep you up to date on the latest information on cancer and chronic disease and on our annual Answers for Cancer Summit.

Volunteer

Extra hands are always appreciated. You can work at home or come join us at our events. Write admin@bestanswerforcancer.org to discuss volunteer opportunities.

Donate

We put your dollars to work! A whopping 90 percent of every donation goes towards Best Answer for Cancer's mission. Yes, that's right. Because we are mostly a volunteer-run organization, only 10 percent goes towards administrative expenses. And every donation is tax-deductible. www.bestanswerforcancer.org/donate.

Health and Wellness Partnership (HAWP)

One of the ways I have approached healing myself of the diseases I have been gifted with is to partner with my physicians. I have explained my approach of addressing my entire life with my Healing Platform, and I have asked for their support in this. I do not challenge them or make demands. I am simply informing. I understand that most of us are of the mindset that our doctors are the leaders in our healthcare programs. However, I also know that nobody cares as much about my life as I do. Most of my physicians over the years have appreciated my approach and my desire to be a part of my own healing and they have valued the fact that I keep them informed.

A friend and another survivor, Ann Fonfa of the Annie Appleseed Project, has joined with me to take this idea up a notch. We have put together the Health and Wellness Partnership (HAWP) as a way to encourage the relationship between physician and patient in order to achieve better outcomes.

The way it will work is that the patient will go to our website and print out three copies of the HAWP, and they will fill in all three copies to take to their next doctor's appointment. www.bestanswerforcancer. org/hawp. At the appointment, they will present the copies to their doctor for discussion and then both the patient and the physician will sign the three copies. The doctor's signature is just indicating that he/she has received it for the file.

- One copy stays with the physician for the patient's file
- One copy goes in the patient's personal records, and

- One copy gets returned to Best Answer for Cancer Foundation. We will report on the number of patients and physicians who get involved with the study.

Eventually, it is our desire to show these numbers to Capitol Hill to demonstrate that patients of cancer and chronic disease want to treat their health holistically.

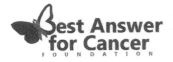 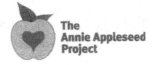

HEALTH AND WELLNESS PARTNERSHIP

An Informal Study on Patient Compliance, Cooperation, and Communication

Dear Doctor: I believe that it is key to my health and healing to address all aspects of my life that might be contributing to the disease. This includes not only the physical manifestations of my disease, but the associated aspects of epigenetics (diet and environment especially), the health of the gut biome and immune system, and the mind-body connection. I may choose additional therapies which are complementary to the therapies agreed upon by my physician(s) and myself, and will keep my physician(s) informed of the nature of those therapies because I respect the doctor-patient relationship and I wish to keep the doctor fully informed. This is an effort to inform my medical professionals and update my medical file. I am not asking my physician(s) to review and assess the effectiveness or safety of listed treatments and I release any physician who has not prescribed or recommended a treatment from any liability merely because I am providing this information to him or her.

With this document, I (Name) *ANNIE. W. BRANDT*

located at (Mailing Address) *ADDRESS*

am informing my physician and/or health management group of components of my personal healthcare that he/she/they may not be aware of or may not be directly participating in. Next to each category, I have listed the personal therapies I am employing at home. It is to be added to my health records file.

My Healing Platform for (disease) *STAGE IV BREAST CANCER*
is as follows:

SPIRITUALITY: *DAILY PRAYER; PRAYER GROUP; WEEKLY LAYING ON OF HANDS*

MIND/BODY: _VISUALIZATION; VISION BOARD; AFFIRMATIONS; MEDITATIONS; NUCALM._

IMMUNITY: _LAUGHTER; WALKING; PET; MUSIC; BELLY BREATHING; ACUPUNCTURE; MEDITATION; AFFIRMATIONS; MELATONIN._

NOURISHMENT: _PALEO DIET INTERSPERSED WITH PERIODS ON RAW, ORGANIC, VEGAN DIET; WILD BLUE GREEN ALGAE; IV VITAMIN C._

DETOX: _VOLLARA AIR & WATER PURIFIERS; EFT; RAW ORGANIC VEGAN JUICES DAILY; WILD BLUE GREEN ALGAE_

LIFESTYLE: _BED BY 9:50 PM; DAILY SUNSHINE. DAILY LAUGHTER; DAILY NUCALM; COUNT BLESSINGS DAILY; BELLY BREATHING_

TARGETED THERAPIES: _IV VITAMIN C; ESSIAC TEA; METFORMIN; FEMARA; IPT; UBI; CHELATION; SARRACENEUM FOOT SPRAY; PECTA-SOL-C; IMMPOWER ER; METATROL; WOBENZYM-N; MEDICAL CANNABIS; POLY-MVA; ARGENTYN 23; NUCALM_

PATIENT: _____
                          Signature

_____   _____
Printed Name   Date

PHYSICIAN: _____
                          Signature

_____   _____
Printed Name   Date

CHAPTER XVIII

Final Thoughts

I am a person who has been given what amounts to a potential death sentence at least three times now, and I have managed and triumphed over each disease. Even when the therapies are contradictory, I have managed to build a tightrope between them to overcome them. Such is the case with ME and MS; one needed exercise, and the other was worsened with exercise.

By the very severity of each of these diseases, I am still a disabled person. I am what doctors call "non-calendar reliable" meaning I cannot keep any kind of consistent schedule. Unlike most people, I have no energy reserves. So when I expend too much energy, I am literally drained and have to take to my bed. I cannot stand for long periods of time or my blood pressure drops. I'm also never sure how I am going to react to public health situations like viruses, etc., because of my dysfunctional immune system. But I am also still very much alive.

What Have I Done With The Life That Has Been Gifted To Me?

Thanks to The Healing Platform that I built, I am living as vibrant a life as it is possible to live. In 2003, I announced to my IPT doctor my plans to create a 501(c)3 nonprofit called Best Answer for Cancer to support IPT and The Healing Platform. Once I examined the process, however, it turned out to be too expensive a prospect at the time because I had just drained my financial resources with the cancer treatments.

My IPT doctor told me about another IPT patient who was starting something similar, Rachel Best. Rachel and I met and decided to join forces. She had begun a project under the umbrella of the National Heritage Foundation. It was called The Elka Best Foundation, and it was named after her mother who died of conventional chemotherapy. The Elka Best Foundation (EBF) was a private organization, with only Rachel as an officer. I became her Assistant Director.

In 2006, Rachel caught an infection in the hospital during a routine procedure. In retrospect, they now think it was MRSA. After three painful months, Rachel died. When I took over the EBF, there was very little money in the bank and we had two paid consultants. I decided to re-create the EBF as an actual 501(c)3 and open it up to both IPT physicians and patients.

Under the umbrella of the Foundation, we opened an online physician's organization called the International Organization of IPT Physicians (later updated to the International Organization of Integrative Cancer Physicians—the IOICP). We also opened a Patient/Survivor Center, where patients could go to share experiences, ask questions, and contribute information.

In 2006, the EBF hosted its first annual IPT conference. Prior to that, the conferences had been small gatherings of interested physicians to discuss case studies. We took it to the next level that year with the announcement of the 501(c)3, the IOIP, and the Patient/Survivor Center. The attendance has grown exponentially over the years, and the conferences are very successful.

EBF experienced positive growth at first. However, it seemed one of our main problems was that the name EBF did not adequately represent what the physicians and the patients were experiencing as they evolved into more integrative approaches. So in 2009, we changed the name to my original idea, Best Answer for Cancer Foundation (BAFC): the best answer for cancer being the one that the individual chooses to address their particular cancer situation.

Since 2009:

- The IOIP became the IOICP, the premier integrative cancer organization in the world.

- As the physicians grew in their use of healing modalities, the IPT Conferences changed their focus to integrative cancer care, and have become the Annual Integrative Oncology Conference; we offer tracks for patients as well as physicians.

- I have become an author: *The Kinder, Gentler Cancer Treatment,* and *Celebrating 365 Days of Gratitude*, and this book!

- In 2010 BAFC sponsored the first clinical study of IPT, a Quality-of-Life Study, under the auspices of Liberty Institutional Review Board (IRB). According to the website www.FDA.gov, "an *IRB* is an appropriately constituted group that has been formally designated to review and monitor biomedical research involving human subjects. In accordance with FDA regulations, an *IRB* has the authority to approve, require modifications in (to secure approval), or disapprove research." Basically it is an oversight committee that monitors clinical trials and studies for the FDA. If you remember, the pharmaceutical industry, which pays for most drug-related studies, has not paid to study IPT since the practice uses just 1/10 of their product and therefore offers no financial benefit to them. BAFC cannot afford to do a clinical trial which typically costs millions. However, we believe that a quality-of-life study will demonstrate that IPT patients experience a kinder, gentler form of treatment than the standard of care.

- I was awarded the March 2012 Legend from RecognizeGood.

- The IOICP has been accepted into the Integrative Medicine Consortium (IMC) as one of its 9 select members. The IMC was founded to bring together the most powerful organizations in integrative medicine in order to collectively change the way medicine is practiced in this country.

- In 2015, we were approved for a new study under Chesapeake IRB: The IPTLD Survival Outcomes Study Using CST and IV Therapies. The study is an IRB-sanctioned version of one completed by Dr. James Forsythe, an integrative medical oncologist in Reno, Nevada. He conducted a five-year study on Stage IV cancer patients using his Forsythe Immune Protocol: chemosensitivity testing, IPT-Lite, IV Vitamin C, Lipoic Acid Mineral Complex, a modified Myers Cocktail, and L-Glutathione. He reports a 71% survival rate after six years and 1000 patients. Our IRB study will chart the survival rates of stage IV patients who choose to do IPT using chemosensitivity testing and the same IV therapies that Dr. Forsythe used. The really exciting thing about this study is that, for the first time, we will have survival statistics for IPT and alternative therapies.

Call it what you will, I love "giving back," and "paying it forward!" I've spoken to thousands of cancer patients since 2006, and I enjoy helping them understand the power of The Healing Platform and creating their own healing platform. Many of them say they receive a sense of empowerment in this process: knowledge is power, and what could be a better weapon against the powerless feeling of a cancer diagnosis? There are also very few people whom I talk to about this book who leave me without feeling an increase in hope, and hope is one of those emotions that have been proven to fight disease.

Time to Build—Key Points for Your Tailored Healing Platform

If you have not already started building your Healing Platform, consider starting now. Here is something you can do right now, to have an effect on your life and to take part in your own thrivorship.

I believe cancer is the true Yuppie disease; it is totally tailored to us. My solution may not be the right solution for you. We are all individuals and therefore the cancer is unique to us and our circumstances. We all need our own best answer for cancer.

As much as possible, do your own research, not only on the internet or in the library, but inside yourself and your life. Yes, it is helpful and much easier to hire a coach to do the research for you.

But consider: Would you just hire a builder, open your front door, and say: "let me know what I should do and how much it is"? If you would not do it with your house, why would you do it with your life? And as far as just going with the flow and doing what most of the people in your family/social circle/church, etc., did, remember the sheep method. Are you really going to go over the cliff to your death with 1498 other sheep just because the first one did?

Another key point is the fact that survival statistics are always measured as five-year survival rates. There is a key reason for this: Because of the damage done to the immune system, the vital body organs, and the healthy cells by surgery, chemotherapy and radiation (see Chapter VII), cancer tends to come back between 6 and 11 years. The survival stats for the pharmaceutical companies, therefore, are best at 5 years.

Find your personal toxins and "dis-ease" and identify your own solutions. You can adjust this platform as needed to change things out or add new things. It is a true "plug-and-play" structure. Remember to change things around from time to time so that cancer does not become immune to any aspect of the platform.

Keep happily and productively busy, but take time to meditate and relax. Remember to do your research, take walks, think about your platform. Keep a notebook of things that you discover, whether you use them or not.

You may be frustrated that I keep saying, "Do your own research." I know that you are fatigued and probably have a good amount of fear around this situation, and you would like me, and others to tell you what to do. As I have said before, cancer is the perfect storm of many factors in your life, and therefore it is unique to you in most ways. If you employ the sheep method and do the "one-size-fits-all" therapy or someone else's recommendation, you will not be addressing all the factors in your perfect storm.

If you consider the "one-size-fits-all" therapy, which is for the most part what is known as the standard of care of surgery, conventional chemo, and radiation, you must consider those dismal survival statistics—purposefully talked of in terms of just 5 years out to mask that treatments are not a cure. The 5-year statistics are just the best-case scenario for the standard of care.

If that does not appeal to you, then you will need to—yes, I'll say it again—do your own research. I really considered it a journey of discovery. I realized I did not know a lot about who I was, what I liked and didn't like, what made me want to *live*. I also realized that there were parts of me that felt like I deserved the cancer and that it would be just easier to die. Somewhere along the road, I read an article that stated that the majority of cancer patients admitted to a feeling of being trapped by life's circumstances with no visible way out of their problems. Many cancer patients I have spoken to over the years confirm this emotion.

I invited my family and my husband at the time to come along with me. It was a fantastic journey—sometimes exhilarating and sometimes very sobering. But always a growth experience.

Your oncologist, in most cases, will not tell you about alternatives and which ones are best for you; you'll just be scheduled for full-dose chemo, radiation, and surgery. Should you decide to pursue alternatives, you may get a lot of pressure from family and friends. Remember to put yourself and your survival first.

The cancer personality puts everyone and everything else first. We all have many tasks in this busy life, but we must remember to put ourselves first. It's like the flight attendant says on the plane: "Put the oxygen mask of yourself first, and then help others around you." The reason for this is that you have about 8-15 seconds before you pass out. How can you help anyone else if you are not around to do it? I had to tell well-meaning people who pressured me to make conventional choices that I loved them, but if I did what they wanted me to do and I died, I would be pretty pissed and I would come back and haunt them. But if I did what I wanted to do and I died, well, that was my choice.

Try to consider this a growth opportunity, not a battle or a fight. Cancer loves the negatives such as conflict, stress, bitterness, resentment, anger, etc. Think about what happens to your body when you hear the word "fight." Instinctively, your muscles tighten up and your body assumes a defensive stance. This type of physical, mental, and emotional reaction creates cortisol, which feeds cancer. And, remember our conversation about the autonomic nervous system? When the "fight or flight" mode is switched on, it shuts off energy to the body systems that are not important to your immediate survival. The two big systems that get put on the back burner are your immune system and your digestive system.

Once I learned this, I refused to have anything to do with campaigns or programs that told me to fight cancer, because I knew I would just be feeding it. Yes, there is anti-cancer value to the initial fight/flight rush, but prolonged stress of this sort is just food to cancer.

So how do you turn this perceived battle-to-the-death around? When most of us get the diagnosis, we see the "picture of cancer" which is that of a very sick person who looks like they are dying. Instead of a battle, consider this a conversation with your body. I looked on it as the cancer dance, and I took the lead. When I realized that the tumors were just manifestations of the dis-ease in my body, I treated them like the messengers that they were. One of my affirmation post-it-notes that remains on my bathroom mirror to this day says, "Thank you, tumors, I got the message: you can go now."

Tests: How to Follow the Cancer

I am not afraid of tests; in fact, I welcome them. We need to put them in perspective. They are just information. Get appropriate testing on a regular basis. How do we know what to do if we do not have information?

That is a good reason to keep the tumor. I know, that sounds like a radical idea. But also consider this: surgery stimulates cancer, causes metastases, and the creation of cancer stem cells. How do you know what is working and not working if you don't have something to measure the results by? You may say tumor markers are good enough, but I know there are false positives and false negatives; my tumor markers showed perfectly normal status when I was diagnosed with end-stage cancer.

Because I read about the dangers of metastases through surgery, I declined to remove the tumors. Yes, this was fairly scary, because our natural inclination is to "get those things OUT of me!" However, the decision to leave them was probably easier for me than for most people. I had been told I only had 3-5 months to live, and I had little reason to doubt that prognosis, taking into consideration all the previous diseases and the dysfunctional immune syndrome. So I was looking hard at the question, "how do I want to die?" and I knew I wanted to die as whole as I could with as much dignity, grace, and quality-of-life as possible. That meant leaving the tumors.

I've never been sorry. Ripping out a tumor does not cure cancer. "We got it all" is not accurate. On the physical level, there are tumor cells and stem cells still circulating in the bloodstream, looking to coalesce into a tumor somewhere else. The immune system is still compromised. Surgery does not address whatever dietary, environmental, emotional, and spiritual challenges we may have that contributed to the cancer.

During my IPT treatments, I did ultrasounds at certain frequencies correlating to the treatment to see what the tumors were doing. If I had not had the tumors, I would have had to wait for the PET scans to see what was going on. Remember, my blood work and tumor markers were completely normal.

Now, I have an annual PET scan. PET scans were pretty much all that was available back in 2001; today, they combine the PET scan with the CT scan. Both use radiation. Dr. James Forsythe tells us the PET/CT scan delivers 600 times the radiation of a chest X-ray. Because of this, it is something to be avoided if possible. I do it once a year because I see that it is worth the risk. The PET/CT scan is my big body measurement; there is no other way for me to see what is going on in my whole body. Dr. Isaac Eliaz gave me a regimen of modified citrus pectin capsules (his product is called PectaSol-C) to take when flying to mitigate the effects of radiation. It is: 4 capsules with the first meal, and 4 every 6 hours of flying. Then 4 capsules 2x/day with meals for 2 more days.

I also have an annual breast MRI, and I have breast ultrasounds about 3-4 times per year. They don't use radiation. As I said, it is good information, and I want to know what is going on in my body.

Let me take a minute to talk about mammograms, which I will never do again. Radiation is carcinogenic. If you have the BRCA gene mutation, for example, getting that annual mammogram is one of the riskiest things you can do because BRCA1 and BRCA2 genes make proteins that act as a tumor suppressor, and they mend breaks in DNA. Faulty BRCA genes are not doing those jobs; they can't help protect us against radiation damage from medical X-rays. And for the rest of us, the reality of mammography for breast cancer screening has fallen woefully short of its promises. A study published in *JAMA Internal Medicine* found that although more women were undergoing regular mammograms, the number of people dying from breast cancer remained the same, and the number of women receiving false positive diagnoses was high.[99] Breast cancer ranks second (after lung cancer) as a cause of cancer death in women in the United States, and the establishment simply didn't promote a good screening technology. Mammography needs to become a dinosaur, and quickly. Dr. Russell Blaylock sums up the numerous problems with mammograms:

> The number of early cancers found by mammograms aren't that many, and 80 percent of lesions spotted in scans are in situ carcinomas, which are considered benign in behavior. If you already have a cancer, in addition to being painful, the crushing compression the breast undergoes during a mammogram can cause

99 Kerlikowske K, Zhu W et al. Outcomes of Screening Mammography by Frequency, Breast Density, and Postmenopausal Hormone Therapy. *JAMA Internal Medicine*. May 13, 2013, Vol 173, No. 9

the cancer to spread. If you have a cancer and you subject it to more radiation by a mammogram, you're going to damage the DNA even more and make the cancer more aggressive. Radiation is inflammatory, and it makes cancers more aggressive and invasive. Women who are at high risk usually have dense breasts, and a mammogram can't read dense breasts.[100]

MRI scans are more accurate, more comfortable. They are also safer because they do not involve radiation, they do not compress the breast, and they can read dense breasts. Thermography, when done properly, can be a good and non-invasive tool for baseline monitoring.

There are so many options out there today for detecting cancer early. Just the different testing and diagnostic methods that are becoming available are exciting. Dr. Rick Davis, a cancer survivor himself, decided that when it came to early detection, we could be doing a lot better. He is an engineer, chemist, medical doctor, and entrepreneur with more than 400 patents and trademarks. Now he wants to revolutionize lab tests, many of which he wants to be available in clinics for more immediate results. He is the CEO of QuickLab™ in Florida and explains his focus:

> Our principal efforts are being directed toward three activities: 1) Selling Hospira's line of IV Fluids & Accessories with a zone-rated delivery guarantee, 2) Providing central-laboratory-based quantitative ELISA testing for serum levels of nagalase and ENOX2 with a 2-day turnaround guarantee, and 3) Developing a proprietary line of Rapid Test Strips & Reader technologies for nagalase and ENOX2 for use in a physician's office.
>
> IV fluids sales are expected to begin in August/September 2016, with the ELISA tests ready by October, and the test strips coming on line in the first quarter of 2017. The ability to quantitatively test nagalase and ENOX2 levels provides clinicians with a powerful and highly cost-effective new tool to screen, diagnose, stage, treat, and monitor cancer unlike anything before. Since nagalase levels measure cellular immuno-competency to fight

---

100 Hubbard S. Can Mammograms Spread Cancer? Newsmax, Oct 1, 2015

cancer, and ENOX2 measures tumor burden, serial measurements of paired tests allow physicians, for the first time, to accurately answer the question: "Doctor, is my treatment working?"

The sheer volume of information about new and better tests can be a challenge to find. One of my favorite new tools and something I recommend to everyone I know—whether they are ill or completely healthy—is *Cancer Free! Are You Sure?* a book by Jenny Hrbacek, a nurse and fellow cancer survivor. As Jenny says:

> This is the "go-to" book for early cancer detection tests which are changing the way the world detects cancer. Americans are led to believe the only way to discover cancer is to wait for a tumor to grow big enough to see it with a mammogram, PSA screening, or PET scan. This is DEAD WRONG. These tests are late diagnostic. You are wasting valuable time because the information comes too late to save you from toxic therapies that may even lead to a recurrence. This book is the road map for how to detect cancer years before standard tests do. If you are in treatment, this book also tells you how to avoid being subjected to the conventional one-size-fits-all cancer treatment. You can find out what drugs and natural therapies will be effective for your specific cancer and tailor a personal program for you.

You can get the latest edition on Amazon or at www.cancerfree-areyousure.com. I am changing my plans to include some of these early-detection tests. I'm curious to learn if any of them can replace the PET/CT scan. My goal is to keep cancer on its toes, not vice-versa.

Keeping Cancer on its Toes

What else can you do to turn the ship around, to become a dance floor instead of a battlefield?

Constantly check your programs and calendars to ensure you have no discernable patterns of therapies to which cancer can build immunities. I really believe cancer can get wise to the damaging values of everything except God and the mind. I did, and do, have therapy programs that have a schedule such as IV Vitamin C 2x/week, but I do my best to change it up somehow with other things so that the cancer is confused.

Don't stand still or settle into a routine where you are a sitting duck. A new friend of mine is a locally famous college football player who has been diagnosed with Stage IV colon cancer. He had some conventional therapy at first but decided that he could not physically handle it and was not willing to spend his last months in that condition. When I met him a month later, I asked him what he was doing for the cancer and he told me he was spending a lot of time with God.

One of my belief systems is that "God is Large and In Charge" (yes, just like it is written there), but I also know that God helps those who help themselves. So I asked my friend, "When you caught the ball on the field and the whole defensive line started coming at you, did you just stand there?" He said "no, of course not." And I said, "So why are you just standing there now?" About three months later, I saw this friend again and he looked better. He said he incorporated some of my suggestions that are in this book and was feeling a lot better.

One of my tenets is to "never let it see you coming." Don't just stand there, and don't be predictable. Be the Emmitt Smith of cancer. (For those of you who are not Dallas Cowboy fans, Smith was a fantastic running back and is now a pro-football Hall of Famer. He was determined to succeed.)

Have you noticed that I do not frequently capitalize cancer? I would also never call it the Big C, and that is not because I am a Christian, or because style books say the word shouldn't be capitalized. I read about the power of emphasis and belief. I will not give cancer any more power over my body than necessary. By making it important in presentation, thought, speech, and action, I am giving it power.

One of my visualizations was to see how really small and powerless cancer was in my body. I would visualize it as so tiny, and getting smaller every minute of every day. Another exercise, especially in the beginning, was to peel the cancer out of my ears (to stop the roar that

I could not hear over) and off my face (to let me see again) and hold it out in the palm of my hand at the end of my arm as far away from my body as possible and say, "I am bigger than you."

Remember not to bury negative emotions and memories. It is important that you process these negatives and come to terms with them; then you can go on to a positive outlook on the issue, memory, or situation. It is interesting to look at studies done on those who survived the degradation and abject misery of Nazi concentration camps in WWII. Viktor Frankl, a survivor who went on to become a world-famous psychotherapist, wrote that those who focused on the importance of finding meaning in life, especially through loving relationships, were more able to overcome the experience. Yet even so, survival came at some emotional cost for many. The term "survivor's guilt" came into our lexicon.

Cancer survivors who have looked death in the face struggle with a version of that also. In my case, why am I a survivor more than 15 years later? Why did I survive while friends and family died? Who was I to survive? I did a lot of research in the library and on the internet. I asked a lot of questions of doctors and every survivor I could find. What makes a cancer survivor?

Some common traits in survivors are that they take control of their lives and they create a method of addressing/changing their lives. It was a confirmation of the approach I had employed throughout my healing journey, and it was an affirmation of me. It made me feel grateful, and an attitude of gratitude is another trait of survivors.

I worked hard over these last two decades to identify, eliminate, and manage the components of my 'dis-ease', and it worked for me. By dis-ease I mean the natural state of "ease" being imbalanced or disrupted. I share this information and process with you, so that you can triumph too. So that you can experience "thriving while surviving."

To properly release the hold cancer has on you, you need to give up things that support and feed cancer, and add the things that are unsupportive of and destructive towards cancer. What do you need to add and what do you need to take away that will clean up your system, boost your immune system, and rebalance your life? How can you stop feeding cancer?

Does any of this sound too complicated or like too much work for you? In a previous exercise, you have imagined the teeter-totter for your immune system. Now imagine the Scales of Justice for your life. Put dying of cancer on one side and on the other side put whatever you think is too difficult to do, like giving up sugar or dairy, or taking on a fresh, organic diet, then make your choice:

Die of cancer or give up _____
(Fill in the blank with things like beer, sugar, cigarettes, etc.)

Die of cancer or start doing _____
(Fill in the blank with things like exercise, detox, colonics, diet, meditation, etc.).

This exercise should be a no-brainer. However, I have actually had cancer patients say to me that they could not give up their candy or their cigarettes, etc. They are no longer with us in this world, but I don't challenge their decisions or yours. I believe this, and I hope you will believe, too:

It's Your Choice
Because It's Your Life

About the Author

Annie Brandt came to be the President Emeritus of Best Answer for Cancer Foundation (BAFC) and the International Organization of Integrative Cancer Physicians (IOICP) from the ground-up: as a survivor of advanced-stage metastatic breast cancer.

After being diagnosed in July 2001 with breast cancer and metastases to the lymph, brain, and lungs, Ms. Brandt was told to "get your affairs in order" and was given three to five months to live. She decided to take a journey on the road less traveled and refused the standard of care: no surgery, no high-dose chemotherapy, or radiation. Instead, she created her own healing platform of holistic modalities that addressed the "dis-eases" in her body, mind, and spirit, and topped it off with targeted cancer therapies.

In 2002, she found Insulin Potentiation Targeted Low Dose therapy (IPTLD or IPT), a simple and elegant targeted cancer therapy: a true Trojan Horse. Eight months later, after adding this targeted cancer therapy to her existing healing platform, her body was cancer-clear.

Ms. Brandt believed other patients should have the option of experiencing thriving while surviving, so she founded Best Answer for Cancer Foundation (BAFC) in 2006. BAFC is a hybrid 501(c)3 nonprofit, comprised of a physicians group (the IOICP) and a general public/patient group.

Ms. Brandt has planned and implemented the International Integrative Oncology conferences since 2006. She has created, organized, and brought to fruition the 2013 ACAM Pre-Conference Integrative Oncology Workshop. At that workshop, she presented the *IOICP Definition of Integrative Oncology* and *Shifting the Cancer Paradigm.*

Prior to the health care industry, Ms. Brandt worked as a Market Research Specialist for Anheuser-Busch Industrial Products Division and as a Systems Engineer for Digital Equipment Corporation (DEC), rising through the ranks to Corporate Information Networking Consultant for the Fortune 100. She became an entrepreneur in the field of Indoor air/water quality consulting, and has owned her own firm in that specialty since 1994. From 1997 to 2004, Ms. Brandt was also co-owner of a "green" design/build company, which was featured in Professional Builder Magazine and won the 2001 Environmental Awareness Award from the City of Austin, Texas for the innovative green complex known as The Villas at Mia Tia Circle.

Ms. Brandt brings this same entrepreneurial, innovative, and pioneering spirit to the field of Integrative Oncology. She has motivated her physicians group, the IOICP, and Best Answer for Cancer Foundation itself, to shift the cancer paradigm from a disease-centered approach to a patient-centered approach, from a one-size-fits-all model to true individualized care for cancer and chronic disease. Ms. Brandt's book, *The Healing Platform*, helps cancer patients discover their own "best answer for cancer." She has co-authored two books: *The Kinder, Gentler Cancer Treatment* and *Celebrating 365 Days of Gratitude.* She is also featured in the book *Cool Careers for Girls as Environmentalists.*

CPSIA information can be obtained
at www.ICGtesting.com
Printed in the USA
FSOW04n0824230217